Neonatal Sepsis *and* Meningitis

Neonatal
Sepsis
and
Meningitis

Alistair G. S. Philip, M.D.

Director, Division of Neonatology
Maine Medical Center

G. K. HALL MEDICAL PUBLISHERS
BOSTON, MASSACHUSETTS

Copyright © 1985 by G. K. Hall & Co.

G. K. Hall Medical Publishers
70 Lincoln Street
Boston, Massachusetts 02111

85 86 87 88 / 4 3 2 1

Library of Congress Cataloging in Publication Data

Philip, Alistair G. S.
  Neonatal sepsis and meningitis.

  Includes index.
    1. Septicemia in children.   2. Infants (Newborn)—
Diseases.   3. Meningitis in children.   I. Title.
[DNLM: 1. Infant, Newborn, Diseases.   2. Meningitis—
in infancy & childhood.   3. Septicemia—in infancy &
childhood. WC 240 P549n]
RJ320.S45P48   1985   618.92′01   84-10873
ISBN 0-8161-2253-9

The author and publisher have worked to ensure that all information in this book concerning drug dosages, schedules, and routes of administration is accurate at the time of publication. As medical research and practice advance, however, therapeutic standards may change. For this reason, and because human and mechanical errors will sometimes occur, we recommend that our readers consult the *PDR* or a manufacturer's product information sheet prior to prescribing or administering any drug discussed in this volume.

Designed and produced by Carole Rollins

Copyedited by Sandra McLean under the direction of Michael Sims.
Typeset in 11/13 Times Roman by Compset, Inc.

CONTENTS

PREFACE

Neonatal sepsis is a world-wide problem that carries a high mortality even in developed countries. Consequently, it is important that all who care for the neonate should be attuned to this problem. An attempt should be made to diagnose and institute appropriate therapy at the earliest possible moment.

The large number of predisposing factors and clinical manifestations associated with this disorder have led many physicians to prescribe antibiotics indiscriminately. Such an approach has tended to produce antibiotic-resistant bacterial organisms, which remain a problem despite the continued development of antimicrobial agents. The incidence of neonatal sepsis seems to have risen in many centers during the past decade, probably in association with improved survival of very immature and other high-risk infants. Therefore, the subject is as relevant as ever, as is attested to by the very large number of articles published on the subject each year. These articles are scattered through many different journals, making it difficult for the individual to distinguish what is really new and important.

This monograph brings together information that should be of interest to obstetricians, pediatricians, family practitioners, infectious disease specialists, and nursery nurses. It is directed towards clinicians at different levels of experience, including those in training. Although I have used many different ingredients, I hope that the essence retains its flavor. For the inquisitive reader, I have provided a representative sampling of relevant references.

During the past decade I have directed my attention to the diagnosis of neonatal sepsis, and emphasis is inevitably placed upon this aspect. The subject of neonatal sepsis (and meningitis), however, is complex and multifaceted, so there are also chapters on incidence, epidemiology, defense mechanisms, clinical presentations, management, and prognosis. Although we have many answers, many questions remain. Continuing investigation in a multiplicity of areas may improve our understanding; but, despite the recent advances in our knowledge, this fascinating subject is likely to remain a challenge for many years to come.

ACKNOWLEDGMENTS

I would like to thank Patricia A. O'Connell, Medical Editor with G.K. Hall Medical Publishers, for initially stimulating me to write about this subject and for later being patient and understanding; Sandra Perry for her cheerful attitude to typing many revisions; and my wife, Elin, for tolerating the inevitable disruptions of daily living occasioned by writing this book.

INTRODUCTION

Neonatal sepsis, or septicemia, may be defined (according to Dorland's) as a systemic disease of the newborn associated with "the presence in the blood or other tissues of pathogenic microorganisms or their toxins"; however, the term is used most commonly to mean the presence of a positive blood culture for bacteria (bacteremia) in association with clinical manifestations of infection. Neonatal meningitis frequently is indistinguishable from sepsis on clinical grounds, may occur concomitantly, and is characterized by infection of the meninges and cerebrospinal fluid (usually documented by a CSF culture positive for bacteria). While the following pages will be devoted to bacterial infection, it is important to remember that some viral infections may be difficult to distinguish from bacterial sepsis.

Despite the proliferation of literature pertaining to neonatal infection, neonatal sepsis and meningitis continue to be major contributors to neonatal mortality and morbidity. Indeed, as a result of significant decreases in other causes of neonatal mortality, neonatal sepsis (and meningitis) has assumed a more, rather than less, prominent role in mortality over the past 20 years.

The reader may find my efforts to summarize what is important regarding neonatal sepsis and meningitis to be presumptuous. After all, in 1971 Pamela Davies illustrated the explosion of interest in neonatal and fetal infection by retrieving 17,147 relevant items on a MEDLARS search of the literature from 1963 to 1969.[1] In preparing this book I did not perform a similar search, because the number of articles published in the last 10 years is presumably even more overwhelming. I have tried to incorporate only those articles from the past decade that seem appropriate to the subject or with which I am particularly familiar. Inevitably, the end result is not a comprehensive review of neonatal sepsis and meningitis; however, I hope that my personal bias does not intrude.

Reference

1. Davies, P. A. Bacterial infection in the fetus and newborn. *Arch. Dis. Child.* 46:1–26, 1971.

O N E

Incidence

Although definitive diagnosis of neonatal sepsis and meningitis usually is based on a positive blood or CSF culture, which normally takes a minimum of 24 hours, a number of other diagnostic tests (to be described in detail later) have been used in an attempt to make an early diagnosis. Because many clinical presentations of neonatal sepsis and meningitis are common to numerous other illnesses, a definitive diagnosis can be quite difficult to make. This difficulty probably accounts for the proliferation of literature; however, the belief that we should be able either to prevent or successfully treat infection of the newborn also contributes to the general interest in this subject. Our frequent failure in preventing or treating infection is a continuing source of frustration. Some of the reasons we fail will be explored in subsequent chapters.

Infection continues to play a significant role in perinatal mortality. When Naeye evaluated the causes of perinatal mortality in the U.S. Collaborative Perinatal Project in 1977, he showed that amniotic fluid infection syndrome accounted for approximately 17% of perinatal deaths, with approximately two thirds being neonatal deaths.[2] On the other hand, Edourd and Alberman suggest that in England and Wales the number of perinatal deaths that were certified as attributable to infection was constant at 1.3% to 1.5% for the years 1968 through 1972 and rose to 1.8% by 1978.[3] Although there seemed to be some absolute decrease from 0.37 deaths per 1000 total births in 1968 to 0.28 deaths per 1000 total births in 1978, because of decreases in other causes of death, the relative percentage increased. Nevertheless, it is apparent

1

that infection remains an important contributor to neonatal deaths—one that should be possible to prevent.

Although improved survival of very low birth weight infants has increased the potential for developing late-onset infection (i.e., occurring 5 or more days postdelivery) in these susceptible infants, the majority of cases of neonatal sepsis and meningitis still seem to occur during the first 2 weeks of life. In 1976 Quie indicated that 75% (53) of 71 babies with meningitis and septicemia became ill within 10 days of birth and nearly 90% of premature, or preterm, infants with positive blood cultures developed signs of septicemia within the first few days after delivery.[4]

The increased susceptibility of preterm infants was first emphasized by Buetow and colleagues in 1965.[5] They found that serial autopsy data showed that the primary cause of death was infection in 10% to 22% of neonates. They collected data on 158 low birth weight infants who fulfilled their criteria for septicemia, which created an incidence of 54.3 per 1000 premature live births (birth weight: 1001–2500 g). The mortality for this group was 50%. The incidence of septicemia in different weight groups was as follows:

Birth Weight	Sepsis Rate
1001–1500 g	164/1000
1501–2000 g	91/1000
2001–2500 g	23/1000

In contrast to these remarkably high figures, McCracken and Shinefield in 1966 estimated the incidence of septicemia to be approximately 1 in 230 live births (or 4.3/1000) in premature infants and 1 in 1200 live births in full-term infants.[6]

Naeye and colleagues noted in 1978 that twins have perinatal death rates caused by bacterial infections of the amniotic fluid that are several times higher than that for singletons (29.4 vs 6.5 deaths/100).[7] Much of this effect may be attributable to the increased incidence of preterm delivery in twins.

In smaller hospitals, considerable year-to-year fluctuation in the incidence and the predominant causative organism of neonatal sepsis and meningitis is likely which makes assessing the incidence for a particular organism difficult. In larger institutions, more accurate estimates are possible. For instance, Baker has shown that the attack rate for neonatal sepsis, meningitis, or both at the Jefferson Davis Hospital, Houston, was between 4 and 8 per 1000 live births in the years 1969 to 1978. The incidence of early-onset group B streptococcal (GBS) sepsis or meningitis in the seventies varied between 1.3 and 4.0 per 1000 live births[8]; late-onset GBS infection seems to have been approximately 0.6 to 1.3 per 1000. This incidence may now be changing as other organisms again become more prevalent.[9-11]

In most centers there are 1 to 3 cases of meningitis for every 10 cases of sepsis. Overall in 1970 showed the overall incidence of neonatal meningitis to be 0.4 to 0.6 per 1000 live births; it was approximately 1.4 per 1000 in preterm infants.[12]

At the Los Angeles County–University of Southern California Medical Center, which has well over 10,000 deliveries per year, the incidence of neonatal sepsis for several representative years is shown in table 1.1.[13] These numbers are similar to those reported from the Yale–New Haven Hospital, where over a 50-year span, the incidence varied between 2 and 4 per 1000.[14] The results of both these studies suggest that more than half of the positive blood cultures were obtained in the first 48 hours after birth. In the author's experience in Vermont, 24 of 50 infants (48%) with neonatal sepsis detected in the first 30 days after birth had the diagnosis made within 48 hours postdelivery.[15,16]

The figures in these studies from the United States are not dissimilar to figures recently reported from Stockholm, Sweden. Bennet and colleagues reported that the incidence of sepsis seemed to be increasing

Table 1.1.
Incidence of Neonatal Sepsis at the Los Angeles County–University of Southern California Medical Center

	1967	1973	1975	1981*
Total live births	10,595	10,301	11,458	6,025
Neonates with sepsis	50	27	35	33
Rate of sepsis (per 1000)	4.7	2.6	3.0	5.4

Source: J. E. Hodgman. Sepsis in the neonate. *Perinatol./Neonatol.* 5(Nov/Dec):45–49, 1981.
*January to May.

Table 1.2.

Changing Incidence of Neonatal Sepsis at the Karolinska Institute,
Stockholm, Sweden

	Incidence per 1000 births	
	1969–1973	**1974–1978**
Neonatal septicemia	1.4	3.1
Neonatal meningitis	0.35	0.41
Mortality from infection	0.23	0.29

Source: R. Bennet; M. Eriksson; and R. Zetterström. Increasing incidence of neonatal septicemia: causative organism and predisposing risk factor. *Acta Paediatr. Scand.* 70:207–210, 1981.

in their hospital (table 1.2) and suggested that this might be caused by a higher rate of survival of highly susceptible low birth weight infants.[11] Data from the Hammersmith Hospital, London, also suggest that the incidence of positive blood cultures is increasing and may be caused by different organisms.[10] From 1967 to 1975, the sepsis rate was 1.6 per 1000 and increased to 5.7 per 1000 in the years 1976 through 1979 for inborn babies. For those infants transferred to the hospital's intensive care nursery (mostly infants of low birth weight), the incidence of 76 per 1000 from 1967 to 1975 increased to 165 per 1000 in the years 1976 to 1979.[10] A similar rate (169/1000) for infants admitted to an intensive care nursery in Iowa City, Iowa, has also been reported for the years 1976 to 1977.[17] Incidence at the Hammersmith Hospital decreased to 65 per 1000 for 1979 through 1982, when 1000 consecutive admissions were reviewed; only 17 infants were found to have sepsis in the first 48 hours.[18]

References

1. Davies, P. A. Bacterial infection in the fetus and newborn. *Arch. Dis. Child.* 46:1–26, 1971.

2. Naeye, R. L. Causes of perinatal mortality in the U.S. Collaborative Perinatal Project. *J.A.M.A.* 238:228–229, 1977.

3. Edourd, L., and Alberman, E. National trends in the certified causes of

perinatal mortality, 1966 to 1978. *Br. J. Obstet. Gynecol.* 87:833–838, 1980.

4. Quie, P. G. Neonatal septicemia. *Antibiot. Chemother.* 21:128–134, 1976.

5. Buetow, K. C.; Klein, S. W.; and Lane, R. B. Septicemia in premature infants. *Am. J. Dis. Child.* 110:29–41, 1965.

6. McCracken, G., and Shinefield, H. Changes in the pattern of neonatal septicemia and meningitis. *Am. J. Dis. Child.* 112:33–39, 1966.

7. Naeye, R. L. et al. Twins: causes of perinatal death in 12 United States cities and one African city. *Am. J. Obstet. Gynecol.* 131:267–272, 1978.

8. Baker, C. J. Group B streptococcal infections in neonates. *Pediatrics in Review* 1:5–15, 1979.

9. Broughton, R. A.; Krafka, R.; and Baker, C. J. Non-group D α-hemolytic streptococci: new neonatal pathogens. *J. Pediatr.* 99:450–454, 1981.

10. Battisti, O.; Mitchison, R.; and Davies, P. A. Changing blood culture isolates in a referral neonatal intensive care unit. *Arch. Dis. Child.* 56:775–778, 1981.

11. Bennet, R.; Eriksson, M.; and Zetterström, R. Increasing incidence of neonatal septicemia: causative organism and predisposing risk factors. *Acta Paediatr. Scand.* 70:207–210, 1981.

12. Overall, J. C. Neonatal bacterial meningitis: analysis of predisposing factors and outcome compared with matched control subjects. *J. Pediatr.* 76:449–511, 1970.

13. Hodgman, J. E. Sepsis in the neonate. *Perinatol./Neonatol.* 5(Nov/Dec):45–49, 1981.

14. Freedman, R. M. et al. A half century of neonatal sepsis at Yale. *Am. J. Dis. Child.* 135:140–144, 1981.

15. Philip, A. G. S., and Hewitt, J. R. Early diagnosis of neonatal sepsis. *Pediatrics* 65:1036–1041, 1980.

16. Philip, A. G. S. Detection of neonatal sepsis of late onset. *J.A.M.A.* 247:489–492, 1982.

17. Maguire, G. C. et al. Infections acquired by young infants. *Am. J. Dis. Child.* 135:693–698, 1981.

18. Placzek, M. M., and Whitelaw, A. Early and late neonatal septicemia. *Arch. Dis. Child.* 58:728–731, 1983.

T W O

Epidemiology

Changes in the Past Fifty Years

One of the most fascinating aspects of neonatal infection is the fluctuation from one decade to the next of the predominant organism causing sepsis.[1] Although some of this fluctuation is undoubtedly the result of the introduction of new antibiotics (e.g., penicillin and methicillin) and antiseptic agents (e.g., hexachlorophene), natural fluctuation is probably as important. Such natural fluctuation has been seen with other forms of infection, both bacterial (e.g., neonatal osteomyelitis[2]) and viral (e.g., influenza[3]).

During the past 50 years,[1] the predominant organism causing neonatal sepsis in the United States has been group A β-hemolytic streptococcus in the thirties,[4,5] *Escherichia coli* in the forties,[6] *Staphylococcus aureus* in the fifties,[5,7] *E. coli* in the sixties,[8] and group B β-hemolytic streptococcus in the seventies (table 2.1).[9] The eighties may go down as the decade when the *Staphylococcus* returned[10,11] or when non–group D α-hemolytic streptococci emerged as an important neonatal pathogen.[12]

It is important to remember that during those periods when a certain organism predominated, other organisms did not disappear. Equally important to keep in mind is that local experience may not reflect national trends and that other nations may have quite dissimilar experiences. For instance, at a time when group B streptococcus (GBS) was the predominant sepsis-causing organism in North America, it was extremely rare in Ethiopia.[13] Further examples of these disparities are

7

Table 2.1.
Predominant Bacteria in Neonatal Sepsis and Meningitis

Decade	Predominant bacteria	Other important pathogens
1930s	Group A streptococci	*Escherichia coli* *Staphylococcus aureus*
1940s	*Escherichia coli*	Streptococci
1950s	*Staphylococcus aureus*	*Escherichia coli* *Pseudomonas aeruginosa*
1960s	*Escherichia coli*	*Pseudomonas aeruginosa* *Klebsiella-Enterobacter*
1970s	Group B streptococci	*Escherichia coli* *Listeria monocytogenes*
1980s	? *Staphylococcus epidermidis* ? Streptococci	

displayed in table 2.2, although the time periods covered are not identical.[1,10,11]

Most Frequent Causative Organisms

An awareness of the most likely causative organism clearly has implications for the choice of antibiotic therapy[17]; the following organisms
are most frequently associated with neonatal sepsis and meningitis:

Sepsis	*Meningitis*
Escherichia coli	*Escherichia coli*
Group B streptococci	Group B streptococci
Staphylococcus aureus	*Listeria monocytogenes*
Staphylococcus epidermidis	

Exposure of the infant to microorganisms can occur (1) before delivery,
as a result of infected amniotic fluid or, less frequently, following maternal bacteremia, (2) during delivery, when contact with organisms in
the vagina or on the perineum may occur, and (3) after delivery, as a
result of exposure to organisms in the infant's environment (generally
transmitted by the hands of the primary caretakers).[18-23] Some organisms are therefore more likely to be associated with early-onset sepsis

Table 2.2.

Most Frequently Isolated Organisms in Neonatal Sepsis by Geographic Location

	Berlin* 1965–1978	New Haven† 1966–1978	Stockholm‡ 1969–1978	Madrid§ 1971–1974	Dallas" 1973–1976	London# 1976–1979
Group B streptococci	27 (23%)	97 (25%)	33 (16%)	—	75 (39%)	7 (6%)
Escherichia coli	42 (36%)	122 (32%)	40 (19%)	39 (17%)	32 (17%)	6 (5%)
Klebsiella-Enterobacter	3 (3%)	56 (15%)	22 (10%)	99 (43%)	14 (7%)	5 (4%)
S. aureus	23 (19%)	24 (6%)	57 (27%)	62 (27%)	9 (5%)	5 (4%)
Haemophilus influenzae	—	11 (3%)	—	—	4 (2%)	—
S. epidermidis	—	2 (0.5%)	26 (12%)	—	—	55 (49%)
Enterococcus	1 (1%)	13 (3%)	8 (4%)	—	38 (20%)	—
Pseudomonas aeruginosa	7 (6%)	9 (2%)	—	7 (3%)	6 (3%)	8 (7%)
Total	118	384	210	230	191	113

*H. Schröder and H. Paust. B = Streptokokken als häufigste Erreger der Neugeborenen Sepsis. *Monatsschr. Kinderheilkd.* 127:720–723, 1979.

†R. M. Freedman et al. A half century of neonatal sepsis at Yale. *Am. J. Dis. Child.* 135:140–144, 1981.

‡R. Bennet; M. Erikkson; and R. Zetterström. Increasing incidence of neonatal septicemia: causative organism and predisposing risk factors. *Acta Paediatr. Scand.* 70:207–210, 1981.

§E. Jaso et al. Neonatal sepsis. *Antibiot. Chemother.* 21:151–155, 1976.

"R. L. Wientzen and G. H. McCracken, Jr. Pathogenesis and management of neonatal sepsis and meningitis. *Curr. Probl. Pediatr.* 8(2):1–61, 1977.

#O. Battisti; R. Mitchison; and P. A. Davies. Changing blood culture isolates in a referral neonatal intensive care unit. *Arch. Dis. Child.* 56:775–778, 1981.

and others with late-onset sepsis.[9] The term *early onset* is often used to describe infections occurring during the first 5 days after delivery; however, in order to implicate intrauterine (i.e., amniotic fluid) infection, clinical manifestations of infection should occur in the first 48 hours. Examples of early- and late-onset organisms are shown in table 2.3.

The enterobacteria (especially *E. coli*) seem to exert their influence throughout the neonatal period, while sepsis—and pneumonia—caused by GBS usually is seen early (although meningitis due to GBS is seen later).[9] Similarly, *Listeria monocytogenes,* although not a frequent problem in North America, is quite common in some parts of Europe and is usually associated with early-onset sepsis but with late-onset meningitis.[24] Exposure to *Staphylococcus aureus* tends to occur after delivery; although colonization may occur earlier, it is relatively uncommon to see *S. aureus* infection in the first 2 or 3 days postdelivery.[25]

Less Common Causative Organisms

The following bacteria are less commonly associated with neonatal sepsis and meningitis:

Sepsis	*Meningitis*
Listeria monocytogenes	*Proteus* spp.
Haemophilus influenzae[30,31]	*Salmonella* spp.[42,43]
Streptococcus pneumoniae[32,33]	*Citrobacter diversus*[44]
α-Hemolytic streptococci[12]	*Acinetobacter calcoaceticus*[45]
Group A streptococci	*Streptococcus pneumoniae*
Group D streptococci[28,29]	*Haemophilus influenzae*[46]
Group G streptococci[34,35]	*Plesiomonas shigelloides*[47]
Serratia marcescens[27,36]	*Neisseria meningitidis*[39]
Pseudomonas aeruginosa[26,37]	
Campylobacter fetus[38]	
Neisseria meningitidis[39,40]	
Yersinia enterocolitica[41]	

Table 2.3.
Frequency of Organisms Isolated in Early- and Late-Onset Neonatal Sepsis

	Yale (1966–1978)*		Addis Ababa (1975– 1978)†	
	< 48 hr (%)	> 48 hr (%)	< 72 hr (%)	> 72 hr (%)
β-hemolytic streptococci	48	14	10	15
Group A	0.5	0.5	1	5
Group B	42	10	0.4	—
Group D				
Enterococci	4	3	5	5
Nonenterococci	1	1	—	—
Nongroupable	0.5	—	4	5
Streptococcus pneumoniae	2	—	—	—
Escherichia coli	26	37	17	25
Klebsiella-Enterobacter	6	23	23	8
Staphylococcus aureus	4	9	5	10
S. epidermidis	—	—	18	21
Haemophilus	5	0.5	—	—
Pseudomonas	1	4	4	—
Proteus	2	2	4	7
Acinetobacter calcoaceticus	—	—	9	5
Citrobacter spp.			3	7
Mixed	4	4	—	—
Other	3	8	7	7
Total number of patients	187	197	260	84

*R. M. Freedman et al. A half century of neonatal sepsis at Yale. *Am. J. Dis. Child.* 135:140–144, 1981.

†N. Tafari and A. Ljungh-Wadstrom. Consequences of amniotic fluid infection: early neonatal septicemia. In *Perinatal infections.* Ciba Foundation Symposium, No. 77. New York: Elsevier-North Holland, 1980, pp. 55–62.

Babies who require assisted ventilation may be at particular risk of infection from "water bugs," such as *Pseudomonas* and *Serratia*, because the equipment uses humidified gases, which require heated nebulizers.[26,27,48] Other equipment can also be contaminated, and personnel can carry virulent organisms.

Because a host of other bacteria have been associated with neonatal sepsis and meningitis, it may be valuable to mention some of those that have become more prominent in the past decade, as they may become the predominant organisms at some future point. Both non–group D α-hemolytic streptococci, mentioned earlier,[12] and group D streptococci seem to be important.[28,29] During the late seventies, there were several reports concerning *Haemophilus influenzae*,[30,31,49,50] which frequently presented with pneumonia, and *Streptococcus pneumoniae* (pneumococcus) was associated with a clinical picture remarkably similar to that produced by GBS.[32,33]

Although the role of anaerobic organisms in neonatal infection has been thought to be underestimated,[51] recent evaluation suggests that this may not be the case after all.[52,53] In a review of anaerobic infections in children, there is almost no mention of septicemia in the neonate[52]; in a prospective study in two nurseries only 3 (0.7%) of 455 blood cultures grew anaerobes compared with 37 (8.1%) cultures positive for aerobes.[53]

Maternal Colonization

Clearly, the most constant source of neonatal exposure to bacteria is the mother. A variety of bacteria are likely to colonize the mother's vagina and perineum, by far the most common being the *Lactobacillus*, but *E. coli* and GBS are also important. Also present, but rarely producing neonatal infection, are yeasts and genital mycoplasmas (particularly *Unreaplasma urealyticum*).[54,55] The recent upsurge in the prevalence of GBS infection in the neonate has resulted in a number of investigations into maternal colonization. Both rectal and urinary tract colonization have been suggested as important reservoirs of GBS[56,57] and special properties of mucosal attachment have been proposed, which may make it difficult to eradicate GBS during pregnancy.[58,59] Interestingly, different ethnic groups may have different rates of carriage of GBS; for example, rates are lower in the Mexican-American population.[59]

An intriguing association of increased water use with decreased amniotic fluid infection was observed in Ethiopia and led Naeye to suggest that we need to do more studies on the role of soap and water in preventing infection.[60] The ability of amniotic fluid to suppress bacterial growth seems to be related to nutritional status.[61-63] Zinc deficiency was suggested as the problem, because the zinc/phosphate ratio appears to be disturbed in amniotic fluid that does not suppress bacterial growth; however, zinc supplementation did not produce amniotic fluid with antibacterial properties.[64] A more recent study noted elevated phosphorus concentrations in amniotic fluid of women with intra-amniotic infection, but no alteration of the phosphorus/zinc ratio.[65]

Although many women are colonized by potentially pathogenic bacteria (e.g., GBS), considerably fewer babies become colonized with the same bacteria and even fewer develop overt infection. Reported prevalence of GBS among parturient women varies from 4% to 29%, but estimates of colonized mothers to infected neonates vary from 50:1 to 100:1.[9] By selective culturing (i.e., limiting cultures to those women with premature rupture of membranes of preterm labor) this ratio was reduced to 20:1 in one study.[66]

Nosocomial Spread

Despite the fact that many preterm infants emerge from an infected environment, the majority of babies are not exposed to significant numbers of bacteria before delivery. On the other hand, most babies acquire bacteria after delivery that will present them with no problem, which constitute "normal flora." Unfortunately, postnatal exposure may not always be to "friendly" organisms, and it is therefore desirable to prevent the acquisition of such pathogenic organisms. One approach is to purposely introduce nonpathogenic organisms to colonize the baby.[67] It is frequently assumed that infants born under unsterile conditions require isolation, as they are more likely to harbor pathogenic organisms. This assumption recently has been proved unwarranted, as infants born under nonsterile conditions were colonized with organisms that were less pathogenic than those found in infants born under sterile conditions.[68]

Little doubt remains that the most important component in preventing colonization or infection with pathogenic organisms is meticulous attention to handwashing.[20,69-71] Under normal circumstances, the use of hats, masks, and even gowns does not seem to be important, provided clean hands and arms are the rule when touching infants. If the baby is to be held, an individual gown or plastic apron should be used. Gowns may inhibit entry into the nursery; conversely, they may convey a false sense of security.[72]

Because we do not always pay close enough attention to hand- and armwashing, a number of nursery outbreaks of infection have occurred that have responded to careful attention to nursery technique.[20,36,37,70,73] In one study, the problem was traced to contaminated scrubbing brushes that were used repetitively.[36] Thus, individually packaged brushes or simple handwashing are more appropriate. The presence of pathogenic organisms may not always be influenced by changes that are instituted; therefore, although it is important to be aware of potential problems,[74] the usefulness of routine bacteriologic surveillance has been questioned.[75]

Again, one might intuitively think that babies nursed under radiant heaters are more likely to become colonized than infants in incubators, but this does not appear to be the case.[76] In some nurseries the frequency of nosocomial, or hospital-acquired, infection has been reported to be very high.[73,77] In other nurseries it may be equally high but may go undetected (or unreported) because minor skin manifestations are regarded as of little consequence. Nevertheless, when certain bacteria predominate, the chances are great that cases of sepsis—and possibly meningitis—will be seen. From a practical standpoint, the most important things we can do to prevent nosocomial spread are to:

1. Wash hands and arms before and after examining any baby: even a perfunctory (15-second) wash seems to be effective[69]

2. Wear a gown whenever a baby is held, and change the gown after direct contact

3. Provide individual equipment for each baby (i.e., stethescope, thermometer, and so on)

4. Avoid leaning on incubators and pieces of equipment
   attached or connected to the baby, particularly during
   rounds when pathogenic bacteria can be transferred from
   one baby's environment to the next

It is important to remember that most infants requiring special or intensive care are immunocompromised to a greater or lesser extent; therefore, sepsis is more likely in these infants if they are exposed to pathogenic organisms.

Important Pathogens

Group B Streptococci

As noted earlier, two different clinical presentations have been described.[9,16] The early-onset disease ($<$ 5 days postdelivery) is characterized by sepsis and pneumonia with high mortality (approximately 55%), which may be considerably higher when it is seen within 24 hours of delivery,[78] particularly when very low birth weight babies are involved.[79] In fact, an apparent decrease in the severity of illness in one hospital was entirely attributable to an increase in the number (and percentage) of term infants affected.[79] Late-onset disease ($>$ 5 days postdelivery) has been characterized by meningitis and comparatively low mortality (approximately 15%).

While early-onset disease is considered to be caused by several different serotypes (Ia, Ib, Ic, II, and III), the late-onset disease is almost always due to type III. Despite this tidy differentiation, such a concept may be an oversimplification.[80] It is important to note that approximately 30% of infants with early-onset infection have had meningitis, which is usually associated with type III.[9] Even in the mid-seventies, a spectrum of disease was being described[81] and more recent evidence suggests that some infants with early-onset infection may have a remarkably benign course,[80] while some late-onset illness is fulminant (personal observations). The differences may relate to the virulence of the particular organisms involved.[80,82] In addition to the serotypes already mentioned, epidemiologic studies may be enhanced by the use of bacteriophage typing, which may distinguish between real and apparent nosocomial spread.[82,83]

Escherichia coli

Despite the recent prominence of GBS, the most important pathogen in the neonate for the past 50 years has been *E. coli* and this organism continues to account for a significant number of cases of neonatal sepsis (see table 2.2). Of great interest is the observation that neonatal meningitis is associated with *E. coli* strains that carry K_1 capsular polysaccharide antigen. For instance, in one study of *E. coli* meningitis, 48 (84%) of 57 strains were K_1 *E. coli*.[84] It also seems likely that this antigen is responsible for enhanced virulence,[85] with both higher mortality and neurologic deficit.[84] In contrast, in infants with sepsis without meningitis only 36% of *E. coli* strains isolated from blood contained K_1 antigen.[84] The meningeal invasiveness of *E. coli* was related to the K_1 antigen,[86] which seems to have properties similar to meningococcal group B polysaccharide antigen.

Listeria monocytogenes

Recent reports dealing with neonatal *Listeria* infection have tended to compare the clinical presentation to the presentation of GBS infection, with early-onset and late-onset forms.[16,87] The early-onset form is considered to be associated with septicemia, and the late-onset form with meningitis.[88]

It is possible that *L. monocytogenes* was overlooked in the past: being a gram-positive rod it may be confused with diphtheroids.[87,89] There is a strong suggestion that *Listeria* may be an important pathogen for both fetus and neonate. *L. monocytogenes* has been associated with abortion and stillbirth as well as neonatal disease.[89–91] In the study of Relier and colleagues, the most frequent presenting clinical sign was respiratory distress (58%, or 31 of 53 cases), while meningitis was seen in only 11%.[24] Both in this study and the study of Ahlfors and co-workers, it was suggested that early warning signs might be maternal fever associated with "greenish discoloration" or meconium staining of amniotic fluid in preterm infants.[92] It is also worth noting that nosocomial transmission has been reported.[93]

Haemophilus influenzae

It was mentioned earlier that a number of reports of *H. influenzae* neonatal sepsis and meningitis appeared in the seventies. The mortality from this infection was very high in these reports. As with GBS, *H. influenzae* may mimic respiratory distress syndrome[31,50] but meningitis is infrequent (table 2.4).[94] Because a large number of affected infants were of very low birth weight, it was suggested that this organism might be capable of producing a septic abortion type of picture, with four of nine babies having birth weights less than 1000 g.[49]

In a recent review of 36 neonates with bacteremia or meningitis—in contrast to older children—only 17% were the result of *H. influenzae* type b.[94] The majority were nontypable, with 38% caused by biotype 4. Of the close to 50 previously reported cases of neonatal sepsis, meningitis, or both, more than 80% had been reported since 1975. The mortality from this infection was 30%, in contrast to earlier reports (see table 2.4).[30,31,49,50,95,96] Recent reports of neonatal or early infantile meningitis have also noted a significant number of cases of *H. influenzae* meningitis,[97,98] which raises questions about appropriate antibiotic therapy.[99]

Staphylococci

Many infants acquire staphylococcal colonization in the first few days after birth, but few become bacteremic. It is uncommon for staphylococci to be acquired in the community; most infants become colonized in the hospital.[100] It was feared that the discontinuation of hexachlorophene whole-body bathing would result in an increase in staphylococcal disease.[70,101] Although the incidence of staphylococcal bacteremia has increased recently, natural fluctuations are the most likely cause.[10,11,102] Bennet and colleagues, however, have postulated that the increase is attributable to the increased survival of highly susceptible low birth weight infants.[11]

One interesting epidemiologic feature of staphylococci is the "cloud-baby phenomenon."[103] In an era when staphylococcal infection was very prevalent, transmittal of staphylococci within the nursery was related to this phenomenon, which seemed to implicate a virus in association with the bacteria. Although the most important mode of trans-

Table 2.4.
Haemophilus influenzae Sepsis and Meningitis

Reference	No.	Sex (M/F)	Birth weight <1500 g	Onset <12 hr	Apparent respiratory distress syndrome	Leukopenia	Positive blood culture	Positive CSF culture	Type b	No. surviving
Nicholls, Yuille, and Mitchell 1975[95]	1	1/0	0	1	1	?	1	0	0	0
Khuri-Bulos and McIntosh 1975[96]	4	2/2	0	4	1	1	4	0	2	4
Courtney and Hall 1978[50]	7	?	5	6	5	6	7	1	1	1
Lilien et al. 1978[49]	9	3/6	8	8	6	?	7	3	1	1
Bale and Watkins 1978[30]	3	2/1	1	3	3	?	3	0	1	0
Speer, Rosan, and Rudolph 1978[31]	1	1/0	0	1	1	1	1	0	0	0
Wallace et al. 1983[94]	10	6/4	5	7	5	3	10	1	1	7
Total	35	15/13	19	30	22	10	33	5	6	13

mission is usually by the hands[70] some babies appeared to be surrounded by a "cloud" of staphylococci. Eichenwald and colleagues likened this cloud to the dust cloud that surrounds the "Peanuts" comic strip character Pig Pen.[103]

Perhaps the most important attribute of staphylococci is their ability to develop resistance to antibiotics. Many of the difficulties encountered in the fifties seemed to be the result of penicillin resistance, but the eighties have yielded multiresistant *S. aureus*,[25] so that we may be poised on the edge of another major catastrophe in neonatal nurseries.

A second important consideration at present is that *S. epidermidis* (coagulase-negative staphylococcus) is now clearly implicated as an important pathogen for the neonate, particularly the very low birth weight infant[10,102,104]; intravascular catheters are a possible additional risk factor.[104] These organisms are also developing multiple resistance, so that if staphylococcal infection is being considered (as it must, in the very low birth weight infant after the first few days) it may be necessary to add vancomycin to the antibiotic coverage.[102]

Candida

Although not usually considered as a cause of neonatal sepsis and meningitis (as it is not a bacterial organism), infection with *Candida albicans* is a potential problem in the very low birth weight infant, those who have been on antibiotics for a prolonged period, and those receiving total parenteral nutrition.[105] This infection is usually referred to as systemic candidiasis and can be extremely difficult to eradicate. The CSF findings with *Candida* meningitis may strongly resemble those of a purulent bacterial meningitis.[105,106] After initially encouraging results with miconazole,[107,108] a more recent report suggests that it is not the drug of choice[109] for systemic candidiasis.

Mycoplasma hominis

Mycoplasma also are not considered bacteria, but need to be considered as potential pathogens when bacterial cultures of CSF are negative, despite CSF findings (cell count, protein, and glucose) suggestive of a bacterial meningitis.[106,110] Although rare, there are reports of meningitis complicated by hydrocephalus[111] and brain abscess.[112]

Citrobacter diversus

Citrobacter diversus is worthy of mention because, although it accounts for a relatively small percentage of all cases of neonatal meningitis, it is frequently associated with brain abscess.[44] A review in 1981 noted that 12 of the 16 neonates with brain abscess in whom a causative agent had been isolated had *Citrobacter* as the isolated bacterium.[106] It was also associated with an outbreak of infection that involved a carrier state of the hands of a nurse who had dermatitis.[113]

References

1. Freedman, R. M. et al. A half century of neonatal sepsis at Yale. *Am. J. Dis. Child.* 135:140–144, 1981.

2. Edwards, M. S. et al. An etiologic shift in infantile osteomyelitis: the emergence of the group B streptococcus. *J. Pediatr.* 93:578–583, 1978.

3. "Influenza." In *Report of the Committee on Infectious Disease,* 19th edition. Evanston, Ill.: American Academy of Pediatrics, 1982, p. 121.

4. Dunham, E. C. Septicemia in the newborn. *Am. J. Dis. Child.* 45:229–253, 1933.

5. Nyhan, W. L., and Fousek, M. D. Septicemia of the newborn. *Pediatrics* 22:268–278, 1958.

6. Silverman, W. A., and Homan, W. E. Sepsis of obscure origin in the newborn. *Pediatrics* 3:157–176, 1949.

7. McCracken, G. H., Jr., and Shinefield, H. R. Changes in the pattern of neonatal septicemia and meningitis. *Am. J. Dis. Child.* 112:33–39, 1966.

8. Gotoff, S. P., and Behrman, R. E. Neonatal septicemia. *J. Pediatr.* 76:142–153, 1970.

9. Baker, C. J. Group B streptococcal infections in neonates. *Pediatrics in Review* 1:5–15, 1979.

10. Battisti, O.; Mitchison, R.; and Davies, P. A. Changing blood culture isolates in a referral neonatal intensive care unit. *Arch. Dis. Child.* 56:775–778, 1981.

11. Bennet, R.; Eriksson, M.; and Zetterström, R. Increasing incidence of neonatal septicemia: causative organism and predisposing risk factors. *Acta Paediatr. Scand.* 70:207–210, 1981.

12. Broughton, R. A.; Krafka, R.; and Baker, C. J. Non-group D α-hemolytic streptococci: new neonatal pathogens. *J. Pediatr.* 99:450–454, 1981.

13. Tafari, N., and Ljungh-Wadstrom, A. Consequences of amniotic fluid infection: early neonatal septicemia. In *Perinatal infections.* Ciba Foundation Symposium, No. 77. New York: Elsevier-North Holland, 1980, pp. 55–62.

14. Schröder, H., and Paust, H. B-Streptokokken als häufigste Erreger der Neugeborenen Sepsis. *Monatsschr. Kinderheilkd.* 127:720–723, 1979.

15. Jaso, E. et al. Neonatal sepsis. *Antibiot. Chemother.* 21:151–155, 1976.

16. Wientzen, R. L., and McCracken, G. H., Jr. Pathogenesis and management of neonatal sepsis and meningitis. *Curr. Probl. Pediatr.* 8(2):1–61, 1977.

17. Eriksson, M. Neonatal septicemia. *Acta Paediatr. Scand.* 72:1–8, 1983.

18. Naeye, R. L., and Peters, E. C. Amniotic fluid infections with intact membranes leading to perinatal death: a prospective study. *Pediatrics* 61:171–177, 1978.

19. Ross, J. M., and Needham, J. R. Genital flora during pregnancy and colonization of the newborn. *J. R. Soc. Med.* 73:105–110, 1980.

20. Markowitz, S. M. et al. Sequential outbreaks of infection due to *Klebsiella pneumoniae* in a neonatal intensive care unit. *J. Infect. Dis.* 142:106–111, 1980.

21. Weindling, A. M. et al. Colonization of babies and their families by group B streptococci. *Br. Med. J.* 283:1503–1505, 1981.

22. Eriksson, M. et al. Bacterial colonization of newborn infants in a neonatal intensive care unit. *Acta Paediatr. Scand.* 71:779–783, 1982.

23. Yoder, P. R. et al. A prospective, controlled study of maternal and perinatal outcome after intra-amniotic infection at term. *Am. J. Obstet. Gynecol.* 145:695–701, 1983.

24. Relier, J. P. et al. Listériose néonatale: a propos de 53 cas. *J. Gynecol. Obstet. Biol. Reprod.* (Paris) 6:367–381, 1977.

25. Perez-Trallero, E. et al. Unusual multiresistant *Staphylococcus aureus* in a newborn nursery. *Am. J. Dis. Child.* 135:689–692, 1981.

26. Fierer, J.; Taylor, P. M.; and Gezon, H. M. *Pseudomonas aeruginosa* epidemic traced to delivery-room resuscitators. *N. Engl. J. Med.* 276:991–996, 1967.

27. Rosenthal, E., and Kohns, U. An epidemic caused by *Serratia marcescens* in an intensive care unit for premature and other newborns. *Deutsche Med. Wochens.* 102:1350–1352, 1977.

28. Buchino, J. J.; Ciambarella, E.; and Light, I. Systemic group D streptococcal infection in newborn infants. *Am. J. Dis. Child.* 133:270–273, 1979.

29. Barikatte, K. et al. Group D streptococcal septicemia in the neonate. *Am. J. Dis. Child.* 133:494–496, 1979.

30. Bale, J. F., Jr., and Watkins, M. Fulminant neonatal *Hemophilus influenzae* pneumonia and sepsis. *J. Pediatr.* 92:233–234, 1978.

31. Speer, M.; Rosan, R. C.; and Rudolph, A. J. *Hemophilus influenzae* infection in the neonate mimicking respiratory distress syndrome. *J. Pediatr.* 93:295–296, 1978.

32. McCarthy, V. P., and Cho, C. T. Endometritis and neonatal sepsis due to *Streptococcus pneumoniae*. *Obstet. Gynecol.* 53:47S–49S, 1979.

33. Moriartey, R. R., and Finer, N. N. Pneumococcal sepsis and pneumonia in the neonate. *Am. J. Dis. Child.* 133:601–602, 1979.

34. Appelbaum, P. C. et al. Neonatal sepsis due to group G streptococci. *Acta Paediatr. Scand.* 69:559–562, 1980.

35. Dyson, A. E., and Read, S. E. Group G streptococcal colonization and sepsis in neonates. *J. Pediatr.* 99:944–947, 1981.

36. Anagnostakis, D. et al. A nursery outbreak of *Serratia marcescens* infection. *Am. J. Dis. Child.* 135:413–414, 1981.

37. Drewett, S. E. et al. Eradication of *Pseudomonas aeruginosa* infection from a special care nursery. *Lancet* 1:946–948, 1972.

38. Torphy, D. E., and Bond, W. W. *Campylobacter fetus* infections in children. *Pediatrics* 64:898–903, 1979.

39. Manginello, F. P. et al. Neonatal meningococcal meningitis and meningococcemia. *Am. J. Dis. Child.* 133:651–652, 1979.

40. Clegg, H. W. et al. Fulminant neonatal meningococcemia. *Am. J. Dis. Child.* 134:353–355, 1980.

41. Shapiro, E. D. *Yersinia enterocolitica* septicemia in normal infants. *Am. J. Dis. Child.* 135:477–478, 1981.

42. Davis, R. C. *Salmonella* sepsis in infancy. *Am. J. Dis. Child.* 134:354–355, 1981.

43. Ohlsson, A., and Serenius, F. Neonatal septicemia in Riyadh, Saudi Arabia. *Acta Paediatr. Scand.* 70:825–829, 1981.

44. Graham, D. R., and Band, J. D. *Citrobacter diversus* brain abscess and meningitis in neonates. *J.A.M.A.* 245:1923–1925, 1981.

45. Morgan, M. E. I., and Hart, C. A. *Acinetobacter* meningitis: acquired infection in a neonatal intensive care unit. *Arch. Dis. Child.* 57:557–559, 1982.

46. Berg, U.; Bohlin, A. B.; and Malmborg, A. S. Neonatal meningitis caused by *Haemophilus influenzae* type C. *Scand. J. Infect. Dis.* 13:155–157, 1981.

47. Pathak, A.; Custer, J. R.; and Levy, J. Neonatal septicemia and meningitis due to *Plesiomonas shigelloides*. *Pediatrics* 71:389–391, 1983.

48. Wheeler, W. Water bugs in the bassinet (editorial). *Am. J. Dis. Child.* 101:273–276, 1961.

49. Lilien, L. D. et al. Early onset *Haemophilus* sepsis in newborn infants: clinical, roentgenographic and pathologic features. *Pediatrics* 62:299–303, 1978.

50. Courtney, S. E., and Hall, R. T. *Haemophilus influenzae* sepsis in the premature infant. *Am. J. Dis. Child.* 132:1039–1040, 1978.

51. Chow, A. W. et al. The significance of anaerobes in neonatal bacteremia. Analysis of 23 cases and review of the literature. *Pediatrics* 54:736–745, 1974.

52. Brook, I. Anaerobic bacteria in pediatric infections. *Curr. Probl. Pediatr.* 11(2):1–40, 1980.

53. Greene, G. et al. Anaerobic blood culture survey in two neonatal intensive care units (abstr.). *Pediatr. Res.* 27:113A, 1979.

54. McCormack, W. M. et al. The genital mycoplasmas. *N. Engl. J. Med.* 288:78–89, 1973.

55. Embree, J. E. et al. Placental infection with *Mycoplasma hominis* and *Ureaplasma urealyticum:* clinical correlation. *Obstet. Gynecol.* 56:475–481, 1980.

56. Anthony, B. F. et al. Genital and intestinal carriage of group B streptococci during pregnancy. *J. Infect. Dis.* 143:761–766, 1981.

57. Wood, E. G., and Dillon, H. C., Jr. A prospective study of group B streptococcal bacteriuria in pregnancy. *Am. J. Obstet. Gynecol.* 140:515–520, 1981.

58. Gardner, S. E. et al. Failure of penicillin to eradicate group B streptococcal colonization in the pregnant woman. *Am. J. Obstet. Gynecol.* 135: 1062–1065, 1979.

59. Anthony, B. F. Carriage of group B streptococci during pregnancy: a puzzler. *J. Infect. Dis.* 145:789–793, 1982.

60. Naeye, R. L. In *Perinatal infection.* Ciba Foundation Symposium, No. 77. New York: Elsevier-North Holland, 1980, p. 262.

61. Shlievert, P.; Johnson, W.; and Galask, R. P. Bacterial growth inhibition by amniotic fluid. VII: The effect of zinc supplementation on bacterial inhibitory activity of amniotic fluids from gestation of 20 weeks. *Am. J. Obstet. Gynecol.* 127:603–608, 1977.

62. Woods, D. L. et al. Antibacterial activity of amniotic fluid. *S. Afr. Med. J.* 55:1059–1060, 1979.

63. Appelbaum, P. C. et al. Studies on the growth-inhibiting property of amniotic fluids from two United States population groups. *Am. J. Obstet. Gynecol.* 137:579–582, 1980.

64. Appelbaum, P. C. et al. The effect of diet supplementation and addition of zinc in vitro on the growth-supporting property of amniotic fluid in African women. *Am. J. Obstet. Gynecol.* 135:82–89, 1979.

65. Gibbs, R. S.; Blanco, J. D.; and Hnilica, V. S. Inorganic phosphorus and zinc concentrations in amniotic fluid: correlations with intra-amniotic infection and bacterial inhibitory activity. *Am. J. Obstet. Gynecol.* 143:163–166, 1982.

66. Pasnick, M.; Mead, P. B.; and Philip, A. G. S. Selective maternal culturing to identify group B streptococcal infection. *Am. J. Obstet. Gynecol.* 138:480–484, 1980.

67. Sprunt, K.; Leidy, G.; and Redman, W. Abnormal colonization of neonates in an ICU: conversion to normal colonization by pharyngeal implantation of alpha hemolytic streptococcus strain 215. *Pediatr. Res.* 14:308–313, 1980.

68. Sacks, L. M.; McKitrick, J. C.; and MacGregor, R. R. Surface cultures and isolation procedures in infants born under unsterile conditions. *Am. J. Dis. Child.* 137:351–353, 1983.

69. Sprunt, K.; Redman, W.; and Leidy, G. Antibacterial effectiveness of routine hand-washing. *Pediatrics* 52:264–271, 1973.

70. Najem, G. R. et al. Clinical and microbiologic surveillance of neonatal staphylococcal disease: relationship to hexachlorophene whole-body bathing. *Am. J. Dis. Child.* 129:297–302, 1975.

71. Davies, P. A. Please wash your hands. *Arch. Dis. Child.* 57:647–648, 1982.

72. Evans, H. E.; Akpata, S. O.; and Baki, A. Bacteriologic and clinical evaluation of gowning in a premature nursery. *J. Pediatr.* 78:883–886, 1971.

73. Goldmann, D. A.; Durbin, W. A., Jr.; and Freeman, J. Nosocomial infections in a neonatal intensive care unit. *J. Infect. Dis.* 144:449–459, 1981.

74. Brachman, P. S. Nosocomial infection control: an overview. *Rev. Infect. Dis.* 3:640–648, 1981.

75. White, R. D. et al. Are surveillance of resistant enteric bacilli and antimicrobial usage among neonates in a newborn intensive care unit useful? *Pediatrics* 68:1–4, 1981.

76. Chang, C. T. et al. Bacterial colonization of infants raised in incubators and under radiant heaters. *Arch. Dis. Child.* 52:507–509, 1977.

77. Hemming, V. G.; Overall, J. C., Jr.; and Britt, M. R. Nosocomial infections in a newborn intensive care unit. *N. Engl. J. Med.* 294:1310–1316, 1976.

78. Quirante, J.; Ceballos, R.; and Cassady, G. Group B β-hemolytic streptococcal infection in the newborn. I: Early onset infection. *Am. J. Dis. Child.* 128:659–665, 1974.

79. Pyati, S. P. et al. Decreasing mortality in neonates with early-onset group B streptococcal infection: reality or artifact? *J. Pediatr.* 98:625–627, 1981.

80. Willard, D. et al. Streptococcies de groupe B en périnatologie: 44 observations. *Nouv. Presse Méd.* 8:2463–2467, 1979.

81. Howard, J. B., and McCracken, G. H., Jr. The spectrum of group B streptococcal infections in infancy. *Am. J. Dis. Child.* 128:815–818, 1974.

82. Boyer, K. M. et al. Nosocomial transmission of bacteriophage type 7/11/12 group B streptococci in a special care nursery. *Am. J. Dis. Child.* 134:964–966, 1980.

83. Band, J. D. et al. Transmission of group B streptococci: traced by use of multiple epidemiologic markers. *Am. J. Dis. Child.* 135:355–358, 1981.

84. McCracken, G. H., Jr. et al. Relation between *E. coli* K_1 capsular polysaccharide antigen and clinical outcome in neonatal meningitis. *Lancet* 2:246–250, 1974.

85. Santos, J. I., and Overall, J. C., Jr. Neonatal sepsis and meningitis—recognition, treatment and prevention. In *Pediatrics update: reviews for physicians* (1979 edition), ed. A. J. Moss. New York: Elsevier, 1979, pp. 285–301.

86. Robbins, J. B. et al. *Escherichia coli* K₁ capsular polysaccharide associated with neonatal meningitis. *N. Engl. J. Med.* 290:1216–1220, 1974.

87. Bell, W. E., and McGuinness, G. A. Suppurative central nervous system infections in the neonate. *Semin. Perinatol.* 6(1):1–24, 1982.

88. Larsson, S. Epidemiology of listeriosis in Sweden, 1958–1974. *Scand. J. Infect. Dis.* 11:47–54, 1979.

89. Shackleford, P. G., and Feigin, R. D. *Listeria* revisited (editorial). *Am. J. Dis. Child.* 131:391–392, 1977.

90. Barresi, J. A. *Listeria monocytogenes:* a cause of premature labor and neonatal sepsis. *Am. J. Obstet. Gynecol.* 136:410–411, 1980.

91. Vawter, G. F. Perinatal listeriosis. *Perspect. Pediatr. Pathol.* 6:153–166, 1981.

92. Ahlfors, C. E. et al. Neonatal listeriosis. *Am. J. Dis. Child.* 131:405–408, 1977.

93. Larsson, S. et al. Listeria monocytogenes causing hospital-acquired enterocolitis and meningitis in newborn infants. *Br. Med. J.* 2:473–474, 1978.

94. Wallace, R. J. et al. Non-typable *Hemophilus influenzae* (biotype 4) as a neonatal, maternal and genital pathogen. *Rev. Infect. Dis.* 5:123–136, 1983.

95. Nicholls, S.; Yuille, T. D.; and Mitchell, R. G. Perinatal infections caused by *Haemophilus influenzae*. *Arch. Dis. Child* 60:739–741, 1975.

96. Khuri-Bulos, N., and McIntosh, K. Neonatal *Hemophilus influenzae* infection: report of 8 cases and review of the literature. *Am. J. Dis. Child.* 129:57–62, 1975.

97. Baumgartner, E. T.; Augustine, A.; and Steele, R. W. Bacterial meningitis in older neonates. *Am. J. Dis. Child.* 137:1052–1054, 1983.

98. Enzenauer, R. W., and Bass, J. W. Initial antibiotic treatment of purulent meningitis in infants 1 to 2 months of age. *Am. J. Dis. Child.* 137:1055–1056, 1983.

99. Fulginiti, V. A. Treatment of meningitis in the very young infant (editorial). *Am. J. Dis. Child.* 137:1043, 1983.

100. Maguire, G. C. et al. Infections acquired by young infants. *Am. J. Dis. Child.* 135:693–698, 1981.

101. Hyams, P. J. Staphylococcal bacteremia and hexachlorophene bathing: epidemic in a newborn nursery. *Am. J. Dis. Child.* 129:595–599, 1975.

102. Baumgart, S. et al. Sepsis with coagulase-negative staphylococci in critically ill newborns. *Am. J. Dis. Child.* 137:461–463, 1983.

103. Eichenwald, H.; Kotsevalov, O.; and Fasso, L. A. The "cloud baby." An example of bacterial-viral interaction. *Am. J. Dis. Child.* 100:161–173, 1960.

104. Placzek, M. M., and Whitelaw, A. Early and late neonatal septicemia. *Arch. Dis. Child.* 58:728–731, 1983.

105. Klein, J. D.; Yamanchi, T.; and Horlick, S. P. Neonatal candidiasis, meningitis and arthritis: observations and a review of the literature. *J. Pediatr.* 81:31–34, 1972.

106. Kairam, R., and DeVivo, D. C. Neurologic manifestations of congenital infection. *Clin. Perinatol.* 81:445–465, 1981.

107. Clarke, M. et al. Neonatal systemic candidiasis treated with miconazole. *Br. Med. J.* 281:354, 1980.

108. Tuck, S. Neonatal systemic candidiasis treated with miconazole. *Arch. Dis. Child.* 55:903–906, 1980.

109. McDougall, P. N. et al. Neonatal systemic candidiasis: a failure to respond to intravenous miconazole in two neonates. *Arch. Dis. Child.* 57:884–886, 1982.

110. Gewitz, M. et al. *Mycoplasma hominis:* a cause of neonatal meningitis. *Arch. Dis. Child.* 54:231–233, 1979.

111. Boe, O.; Diderichsen, J.; and Matre, R. Isolation of *Mycoplasma hominis* from cerebrospinal fluid. *Scand. J. Infect. Dis.* 5:285–288, 1973.

112. Siber, G. R. et al. Neonatal central nervous system infection due to *Mycoplasma hominis. J. Pediatr.* 90:625–627, 1977.

113. Parry, M. F.; Hutchinson, J. H.; and Brown, N. A. Gram negative sepsis in neonates: a nursery outbreak due to hand carriage of *Citrobacter diversus. Pediatrics* 65:1105–1109, 1980.

THREE

Defense Mechanisms and Deficiencies

Infants at Particular Risk

As stated in chapter 1, all neonates apparently are at greater risk of systemic infection than are older individuals but some are more susceptible than others.

Premature infants were the focus of one major review of neonatal sepsis.[1] The study showed that such infants are particularly susceptible to infection, with incidence figures as high as 1 in 6 infants with birth weight less than 1500 g, compared with incidence figures of 1 to 3 per 1000 for all neonates (see chapter 1). In a more recent study evaluating a possible change in infant mortality in group B streptococcal (GBS) infection, the very low birth weight infant was shown to have an enormously increased risk of dying compared with heavier babies.[2] Not only is the very low birth weight infant at increased risk of acquiring infection, he or she is also at increased risk of succumbing to such infection.

The increased susceptibility of the low birth weight infant is primarily believed to be the result of immature defense mechanisms, because the infant is born prematurely. There also seem to be differences, however, in infants born small for gestational age, who are either at or close to term. Histologic studies of growth-retarded infants who died showed that the spleen and thymus seemed to be more affected than most other organs.[3] Evidence has also been presented that infants who were small for gestational age may have a lack of T-lymphocytes, both at birth and during the first months after birth,[4] which may contribute to an increased susceptibility to infection.

An old observation that is still noted in present-day series of neonatal sepsis is that male infants are more likely to acquire and succumb to infection in an approximate ratio of 2:1.[5-7] The exact reasons for this enhanced male susceptibility are still unclear and one large series from Spain showed no sex predilection[8]; however, some protection against infection, which seems to be mediated through antibody production,[6] apparently is conferred by the extra X chromosome in females. The more recent observation of an increased risk of GBS infection in twins is also unexplained.[9,10]

Two other small groups of infants have been found to be particularly susceptible to infection and may provide insights into the general mechanisms of defense. The first group, infants with galactosemia, seem to be particularly prone to neonatal sepsis caused by *Escherichia coli*. During a 12-year period, 35 infants with galactosemia were detected by routine screening. Ten of them developed systemic infection and all nine bacteremic babies died despite therapy.[11] In almost every case, the causative organism was *E. coli*, which would not have been anticipated, particularly because these cases were discovered in an era when GBS were predominant. Early diagnosis and treatment of the galactosemia may prevent this form of sepsis, which was most common in neonates aged 1 to 2 weeks.[11]

The second group of infants at risk are those given parenteral iron. In a study from New Zealand, the incidence of neonatal sepsis was 20 times greater in a group of neonates given routine intramuscular iron dextran.[12] This impaired immunity again increased susceptibility to *E. coli*. Administration of iron seems to alter transferrin levels, which may play a role in altering phagocytosis—although this did not seem to be the situation in one study.[13] Because bacteria require iron to proliferate, an excess of iron possibly may enhance bacterial growth and tip the balance.[14] In vitro studies have shown a decrease in bacteriostasis.[13]

Physical Factors

Any open wound is a potential source of access to the bloodstream. This tenet is certainly true of circumcision[15]; the cut end of the umbilical cord may also be considered an example of such a wound. Attempts to prevent colonization of the umbilical cord have resulted in a number of different methods of cord care. Triple dye, hexachlorophene, silver sulfadiazine, and bacitracin (among others) have all been used to minimize bacterial colonization.[16,17] Delayed separation of the umbilical cord recently has been associated with widespread infection, but this may be caused by immunodeficiency rather than umbilical cord infection.[18-20]

In addition to the protective effect of skin itself, the layer of vernix caseosa may also provide protection, although it does not appear to have specific antibacterial properties.[21] Vernix caseosa may be better left on neonates because of the mechanical obstruction it provides to bacterial passage.[21]

Antibodies

In order to clear invading microorganisms from the body, several different mechanisms are involved, all of which seem to be imperfectly developed in the neonate. One of the most important defense mechanisms is the presence or production of antibodies, which are also called immunoglobulins. Most newborns have some deficiency of immunoglobulins because the placenta may allow passage of immunoglobulin G across it, but not other immunoglobulins. Originally considered to be a function of smaller molecular size, passage of IgG is now known to be an active transport mechanism.[22] The end result is that maternal antibodies that belong to the IgG group may provide protection in the neonate, but there is inevitably a deficiency of IgM antibodies. Among the principal antibodies belonging to the IgM group are those that combat *E. coli*. This deficiency accounts in part for the particular susceptibility of the neonate to this organism. Another important consideration is that the transfer of IgG seems to increase with advancing gestational age; therefore, considerably lower levels of IgG are seen in very preterm infants compared with levels in term infants.[23,24] These depressed levels may contribute to the increased susceptibility to infection of preterm infants.

The evidence relating to the susceptibility of some neonates to GBS infection is even more striking than that for *E. coli*. Although antibodies to GBS are predominantly IgG, susceptibility of babies to the various subtypes—Ia, Ib, Ic, II, and III—seems to be closely linked to the presence (or absence) of specific antibody in their mothers and hence in their babies.[25-27] For instance, a mother may have antibody to type II organisms, but this provides no protection for either mother or child against type III organisms. In the study of Vogel and colleagues, 200 consecutive pregnant women in an urban obstetric screening clinic were evaluated together with 108 women with GBS vaginal colonization.[25] Antibody was detected in the clinic population in 26% against serotype Ia, 52% against Ib, 82% against II, and 45% against III. Only 9% had antibody against all four GBS types. In 54 women whose infants developed sepsis, meningitis, or both the prevalence of antibody against the specific serotypes responsible was considerably lower than for the noninfected groups. (Two infected infants had serotype Ia, 8 had Ib, 4 had II, and 40 had III).

Extensive investigation has shown that neonates may fail to produce specific antibody against GBS despite overt infection followed by recovery. Baker and co-workers showed very little (if any) response in 85 infants who survived systemic GBS infection caused by serotype III, whereas each of 5 women with postpartum bacteremia produced high levels of antibody.[27] Although other organisms have not been studied as carefully, it is reasonably clear that although lack of antibody may predispose to infection, production of antibody is not essential for recovery. On the other hand, administration of blood containing specific antibody (either simple transfusion or exchange transfusion[28,29]) may enhance the chances of survival. It is also possible that modified immune serum globulin could be valuable, if donors could be suitably selected.[30]

If we now return to the general topic of immunoglobulins in neonatal infection, there is accumulating evidence that different subtypes of IgG may be more important than others. It has been noted that IgG1 as well as IgG3 is synthesized earlier than IgG2 and IgG4 and reaches adult levels earlier (6 months vs 24 months).[31]

Two other important observations were made many years ago: (1) the fetus is capable of producing immunoglobulins and other proteins at a very early stage of development and (2) the neonate can respond to appropriate stimuli from birth onward, albeit slowly and perhaps selectively.[32,33] The latter point was first noted in an unusual "experiment of nature" when an infant born to an agammaglobulinemic mother was available for study.[32] In a more recent, similar observation, immunoglobulins remained low and antibodies to immunizing antigens appeared late.[34] This pattern suggests "that transplacental maternal antibodies play little or no role in modulating newborn IgG production and that the delays in achieving normal levels of IgG are probably due to the immaturity of newborn B lymphocytes."[34]

Lymphocytes

Not long ago the neonate was considered "immunologically null," but there has been an explosion of knowledge in immunology in general and in neonatal immunology in particular.[35] For instance, in a 1976 review there is no mention of the various types of T cells. They are lumped together as T-lymphocytes.[36] Although the subject is becoming increasingly complex, we need to know something about lymphocyte function, particularly as it relates to neonatal infection.[31] Despite the fact that "demonstrable immune function is present in all viable infants," this immune response is almost certainly immature in most neonates.[35] The production of antibodies (i.e., humoral immunity) is largely under the influence of B cells, and cell-mediated immunity is a T-cell function. As in adult blood, almost 80% of the lymphocytes are T-lymphocytes and, although B-lymphocytes make up a percentage similar to that found in adults, there is a significant reduction in their activity (table 3.1). In addition, natural killer cells seem to be greatly decreased in number, although their function may be intact. Both the number and activity of suppressor T cells are increased in cord blood lymphocytes, and the activity of B cells seems to be inhibited by suppressor T cells. This increased activity of suppressor T cells before birth probably contributes to inhibition of interaction between maternal and fetal cells. After birth, as suppressor T-cell activity decreases, B-cell activity increases and antibody (immunoglobulin) production im-

Table 3.1.
Lymphocytes in Cord and Adult Blood

Type of lymphocyte	Cord blood	Adult blood
T-lymphocytes	80%	80%
B-lymphocytes	5–8%	4–7%
Natural killer cells	1%	3–15%
Ratio of helper T cell to suppressor T cell	1:1	2:1

Modified from W. A. Hitzig. T- and B- lymphocyte systems and their function in premature and full-term neonates. In *Diagnostics in perinatal infections*. Marburg, West Germany: Behring Diagnostica Symposium, May 1983.

proves. Because there is little exposure of most neonates to bacterial antigens in utero, the major stimulus—antigen drive—to antibody production by the B cells is lacking. Response to antigenic stimulation (i.e., to different bacterial antigens) can be quite variable, which may account for both general and individual susceptibility.[36]

As noted earlier, the small for gestational age infant may have a partial lack of T-lymphocytes.[4] Using newer techniques such as monoclonal antisera and a fluorescent-activated cell sorter, total T cells, helper and inducer T lymphocytes, as well as B cells were all deficient in number in small for gestational age infants compared with their term and preterm appropriate for gestational age counterparts.[37] All newborn infants had a highly significant increase in absolute numbers of both helper and suppressor T-lymphocytes compared with normal adults.[37]

Phagocytosis

Neonatal polymorphonuclear (PMN) leukocytes seem quite capable of adequate phagocytosis, provided everything else that contributes to this function is in place. For instance, it has been suggested that PMNs do not adequately phagocytose in the absence of chemotactic factor or in the absence of various opsonins (principally complement). It has also been suggested that stressed or infected neonates have impaired bactericidal activity[38] and that the method of delivery may play a role in leukocyte function, with decreased function seen following vaginal delivery or cesarean section with labor.[39] Any deficiency of PMNs, however, seems to be attributable to a deficiency in the amount of the other substances that prepare bacteria for engulfment by the leukocyte.[40]

Despite this capability to phagocytose, it should be pointed out that the leukocyte response to infection is quite variable. The ability of neutrophils to migrate appears to be compromised in neonates.[41] In severe, overwhelming infection, leukopenia—and more specifically neutropenia—is the rule rather than the exception. The neutrophil storage pool in the bone marrow may rapidly become depleted, with an accompanying increase in the ratio of immature to total neutrophils in the peripheral blood, and eventually a more or less complete agranulocytosis.[42,43]

An additional complicating factor in phagocytosis can be the presence of jaundice. Bilirubin has been noted to inhibit the hexose-monophosphate-shunt activity of phagocytes. Because this activity is an important prerequisite for killing bacteria, jaundice may contribute to the increased susceptibility of the neonate to bacterial infection.[44]

Complement

Low levels of human complement may be seen in the presence of infection, because of increased utilization in the immune response.[45] In the newborn levels of complement usually are considerably lower than in the adult, particularly in preterm infants.[46] The ability to produce complement may start as early as 8 weeks of fetal life,[47] seems to continue throughout fetal life, and gradually increases in the first few months after birth.[48] Whether or not the lower levels contribute to the increased susceptibility of neonates (particularly preterm infants) to infection is not completely clear,[47,48] but lower levels of complement were observed in infected infants.[46] Both classical and alternative pathway activation sequences appear to be deficient.[49,50]

Complement factors are apparently the most important chemotactic and opsonic factors.[35,36] The ability to remove bacteria, especially *E. coli,* from the bloodstream may be determined by both the presence of complement and whether or not the organism is encapsulated. Encapsulated organisms are relatively complement-resistant, because the capsule protects deep somatic antigen structures from activating the alternative complement pathway.[51] A deficiency of complement seems to be the limiting factor in neonatal phagocytosis. As stated earlier, the preparation of bacteria for ingestion by the leukocyte is deficient rather than the act of phagocytosis itself. It is also of interest that the ninth component of complement, C9, although present in low concentration in cord blood, seems to act as an acute-phase reactant after exogenous stimulation.[52]

Acute-Phase Proteins

It has been well demonstrated that infants have the ability to respond to bacterial sepsis with an increase in several acute-phase proteins, or reactants (see chapter 8); however, there is limited information on the function of acute-phase proteins at all ages, including the neonate. It is known that most proteins are present in decreased amounts in the neonate, when compared with levels in the adult or older child. This is true for both haptoglobin[53] and α_1-acid glycoprotein (orosomucoid)[54,55] among the acute-phase proteins, as well as for IgM.[56] C-reactive protein is not normally present in significant amounts in either adults or neonates.[57] There are data to show that C-reactive protein may play a role in phagocytosis[58,59] and may stimulate the complement pathway.[60] Modification of the function of lymphocytes has been reported with α_1-acid glycoprotein,[61] and haptoglobin may have a bacteriostatic role by binding free iron, which can enhance bacterial growth.[62] Some limited experience suggests that failure to produce adequate amounts of these acute-phase proteins is associated with decreased survival in neonates with sepsis.[54,63] Whether the infant with overwhelming sepsis fails to respond, or whether the failure to produce adequate amounts of acute-phase proteins results in uncontrollable sepsis, is uncertain.

Fibronectin

Formerly called cold insoluble globulin, fibronectin is a high molecular weight glycoprotein that seems to have nonspecific opsonic properties and aids in clearing bacteria as well as enhancing immune function of phagocytes (both mononuclear and polymorphonuclear).[64]

Recent evidence supports the idea that low birth weight infants in particular have low levels of fibronectin.[65,66] These levels increase with both increasing birth weight and increasing postnatal age. In some infants with sepsis, particularly low levels have been demonstrated early in the course of infection, which increase during clinical improvement.[67] It seems likely that decreased levels of fibronectin predispose neonates to sepsis, but that lower levels with sepsis might be the result of increased consumption rather than decreased availability.

Experimental evidence indicates that addition of sufficient purified fibronectin to cord plasma to achieve levels in the normal adult range can increase opsonic activity.[68] Whether or not this has practical implications in the treatment of neonatal sepsis remains to be elucidated.

References

1. Buetow, K. C.; Klein, S. W.; and Lane, R. B. Septicemia in premature infants. *Am. J. Dis. Child.* 110:29–41, 1965.

2. Pyati, S. P. et al. Decreased mortality in neonates with early-onset group B streptococcal infection: reality or artifact? *J. Pediatr.* 98:625–627, 1981.

3. Naeye, R. L.; Blanc, W.; and Paul, C. Effects of maternal nutrition on the human fetus. *Pediatrics* 52:494–503, 1973.

4. Chandra, R. K. Serum thymic hormone activity and cell-mediated immunity in healthy neonates, preterm infants and small-for-gestational age infants. *Pediatrics* 67:407–411, 1981.

5. Nyhan, W. L., and Fousek, M. D. Septicemia of the newborn. *Pediatrics* 22:268–278, 1958.

6. Washburn, T. C.; Medearis, D. N., Jr.; and Childs, B. Sex differences in susceptibility to infections. *Pediatrics* 35:57–64, 1965.

7. Tafari, N., and Ljungh-Wadstrom, A. Consequences of amniotic fluid infection: early neonatal septicemia. In *Perinatal infections,* Ciba Foundation Symposium, No. 77. New York: Elsevier, 1980, pp. 55–62.

8. Jaso, E. et al. Neonatal sepsis. *Antibiot. Chemother.* 21:151–155, 1976.

9. Pass, M. A.; Khare, S.; and Dillon, H. C., Jr. Twin pregnancies: incidence of group B streptococcal colonization and disease. *J. Pediatr.* 97:635–637, 1980.

10. Edwards, M. S.; Jackson, C. V.; and Baker, C. J. Increased risk of group B streptococcal disease in twins. *J.A.M.A.* 245:2044–2046, 1981.

11. Levy, H. L. et al. Sepsis due to *Escherichia coli* in neonates with galactosemia. *N. Engl. J. Med.* 297:823–825, 1977.

12. Barry, D. M. J., and Reeve, A. W. Increased incidence of gram-negative neonatal sepsis with intramuscular iron administration. *Pediatrics* 60:908–912, 1977.

13. Becroft, D. M. O.; Dix, M. R.; and Farmer, K. Intramuscular iron-dextran and susceptibility of neonates to bacterial infections: in vitro studies. *Arch. Dis. Child.* 52:778–781, 1977.

14. Bullen, J. J. The significance of iron in infection. *Rev. Infect. Dis.* 3:1127–1136, 1981.

15. Cleary, T. G., and Kohl, S. Overwhelming infection with group B β-hemolytic streptococcus associated with circumcision. *Pediatrics* 64:301–303, 1979.

16. Wald, E. R.; Snyder, M. J.; and Gutberlet, R. L. Group B beta-hemolytic streptococcal colonization: acquisition, persistence and effect of umbilical cord treatment with triple dye. *Am. J. Dis. Child.* 131:178–180, 1977.

17. Barrett, F. F.; Mason, E. O.; and Fleming, D. Effect of three cord-care regimens on bacterial colonization of normal newborn infants. *J. Pediatr.* 94:796–800, 1979.

18. Hayward, A. R. et al. Delayed separation of the umbilical cord, widespread infections, and defective neutrophil mobility. *Lancet* 1:1099–1101, 1979.

19. Bissenden, J. G. et al. Delayed separation of the umbilical cord, severe widespread infections and immunodeficiency. *Arch. Dis. Child.* 56:397–399, 1981.

20. Bowen, T. J. et al. Severe recurrent bacterial infections associated with defective adherence and chemotaxis in two patients with neutrophils deficient in a cell-associated glycoprotein. *J. Pediatr.* 101:932–940, 1982.

21. Joglekar, V. M. Barrier properties of vernix caseosa. *Arch. Dis. Child.* 55:817–819, 1980.

22. Gitlin, D. et al. The selectivity of the human placenta in the transfer of plasma proteins from mother to fetus. *J. Clin. Invest.* 43:1938–1951, 1964.

23. Stiehm, E. R. Fetal defense mechanisms. *Am. J. Dis. Child.* 129:438–443, 1975.

24. Hobbs, J. R., and Davis, J. A. Serum γ-globulin levels and gestational age in premature babies. *Lancet* 1:757–759, 1967.

25. Vogel, L. C. et al. Prevalence of type-specific group B streptococcal antibody in pregnant women. *J. Pediatr.* 96:1047–1051, 1980.

26. Christensen, K. K. et al. Quantitation of serum antibodies to surface antigens of group B streptococci type Ia, Ib and III: low antibody levels in mothers of neonatally infected infants. *Scand. J. Infect. Dis.* 12:105–110, 1980.

27. Baker, C. J.; Edwards, M. S., and Kasper, D. L. Role of antibody to native type III polysaccharide of group B streptococcus in infant infection. *Pediatrics* 68:544–549, 1981.

28. Shigeoka, A.; Hall, R. T.; and Hill, H. R. Blood transfusion in group B streptococcal sepsis. *Lancet* 1:636–638, 1978.

29. Vain, N. E. et al. Role of exchange transfusion in the treatment of severe septicemia. *Pediatrics* 66:693–697, 1980.

30. Santos, J. I. et al. Protective efficacy of a modified immune serum globulin in experimental group B streptococcal infection. *J. Pediatr.* 99:873–879, 1981.

31. Hitzig, W. A. T- and B-lymphocyte systems and their function in premature and full-term neonates. Significance in perinatal infectious diseases. In *Diagnostics in perinatal infections.* Marburg, West Germany: Behring Diagnostica Symposium, May 1983.

32. Holland, N., and Holland, P. Immunological maturation of an infant of an agammaglobulinemic mother. *Lancet* 2:1152–1156, 1966.

33. Gitlin, D., and Biasucci, A. Development of IgG, IgA, IgM, β_1 C/βIA, $C^1$1 esterase inhibitor, ceruloplasmin, transferrin, hemopexin, haptoglobin, fibrinogen, plasminogen, α_1-antitrypsin, orosomucoid, β-lipoprotein, α_2-macroglobulin and pre-albumin in the human conceptus. *J. Clin. Invest.* 48:1433–1446, 1969.

34. Kobayashi, R. H.; Hyman, C. J.; and Stiehm, E. R. Immunologic maturation in an infant born to a mother with agammaglobulinemia. *Am. J. Dis. Child.* 134:942–944, 1980.

35. Miller, M. E. Host defenses in the human neonate. *Pediatr. Clin. North Am.* 24:413–423, 1977.

36. Harris, M. B. Neonatal host-defense mechanisms. *Pediatr. Ann.* 5:86–93, 1976.

37. Thomas, R. M., and Linch, D. C. Identification of lymphocyte subsets in the newborn using a variety of monoclonal antibodies. *Arch. Dis. Child.* 58:34–38, 1983.

38. Shigeoka, A. D.; Santos, J. I.; and Hill, H. R. Functional analysis of neutrophil granulocytes from healthy, infected and stressed neonates. *J. Pediatr.* 95:454–460, 1979.

39. Frazier, J. P. et al. Leukocyte function in healthy neonates following vaginal and cesarean section delivery. *J. Pediatr.* 101:269–272, 1982.

40. Harris, M. C. et al. Phagocytosis of group B streptococcus by neutrophils from newborn infants. *Pediatr. Res.* 17:358–361, 1983.

41. Christensen, R. D., and Rothstein, G. Efficiency of neutrophil migration in the neonate. *Pediatr. Res.* 14:1147–1149, 1980.

42. Christensen, R. D., and Rothstein, G. Exhaustion of mature marrow neutrophils in neonates with sepsis. *J. Pediatr.* 96:316–318, 1980.

43. Christensen, R. D.; Bradley, P. P.; and Rothstein, G. The leukocyte left shift in clinical and experimental neonatal sepsis. *J. Pediatr.* 98:101–105, 1981.

44. Thong, Y. H., and Rencis, V. Bilirubin inhibits hexose-monophosphate shunt activity of phagocytosing neutrophils. *Acta Paediatr. Scand.* 66:757–759, 1977.

45. Levy, D. L., and Arquembourg, P. C. Maternal and cord blood complement activity: relationship to premature rupture of the membranes. *Am. J. Obstet. Gynecol.* 139:38–40, 1981.

46. Drew, J. H., and Arroyave, C. M. The complement system of the newborn infant. *Biol. Neonate* 37:209–217, 1980.

47. Adinolfi, M. Human complement: onset and site of synthesis during fetal life. *Am. J. Dis. Child.* 131:1015–1023, 1977.

48. Davis, C. A.; Vallota, E. H.; and Forristal, Jr. Serum complement levels in infancy: age related changes. *Pediatr. Res.* 13:1043–1046, 1979.

49. Adamkin, D. et al. Activity of the alternative pathway of complement in the newborn infant. *J. Pediatr.* 93:604–608, 1978.

50. Strunk, R. C.; Fenton, L. J.; and Gaines, J. A. Alternative pathway of complement activation in full-term and premature infants. *Pediatr. Res.* 13:641–643, 1979.

51. Wientzen, R. L., Jr., and McCracken, G. H., Jr. Pathogenesis and management of neonatal sepsis and meningitis. *Curr. Probl. Pediatr.* 8(2):1–61, 1977.

52. Lehner, T., and Adinolfi, M. Acute phase proteins, C9, factor B, and lysozyme in recurrent oral ulceration and Behçet's syndrome. *J. Clin. Pathol.* 33:269–275, 1980.

53. Salmi, T. T. Haptoglobin levels in the plasma of newborn infants: with special reference to infections. *Acta Paediatr. Scand.* Suppl. 241:1–55, 1973.

54. Sann, L. et al. Serum orosomucoid concentration in newborn infants. *Eur. J. Pediatr.* 136:181–185, 1981.

55. Philip, A. G. S., and Hewitt, J. R. α_1-Acid glycoprotein in the neonate with and without infection. *Biol. Neonate* 43:118–124, 1983.

56. Haider, S. A. Serum IgM in diagnosis of infection in the newborn. *Arch. Dis. Child.* 47:382–393, 1972.

57. Pepys, M. B. C-reactive protein fifty years on. *Lancet* 1:653–657, 1981.

58. Kindmark, C. O. Stimulating effect of C-reactive protein on phagocytosis of various species of pathogenic bacteria. *Clin. Exp. Immunol.* 8:941–948, 1971.

59. Mold, C. et al. C-reactive protein is protective against *Streptococcus pneumoniae* infection in mice. *J. Exp. Med.* 154:1703–1708, 1981.

60. Gewurz, H. Biology of C-reactive protein and the acute phase response. *Hosp. Pract.* 17:67–81, 1982.

61. Chiu, K. M. et al. Interactions of alpha$_1$-acid glycoprotein with the immune system. I. Purification and effects upon lymphocyte responsiveness. *Immunology* 32:997–1005, 1977.

62. Eaton, J. W. et al. Haptoglobin: a natural bacteriostat. *Science* 215:691–693, 1982.

63. Philip, A. G. S. The protective role of acute phase reactants in neonatal sepsis. *Acta Paediatr. Scand.* 68:481–483, 1979.

64. Mosesson, M. W., and Amrani, O. L. The structure and biological activities of plasma fibronectin. *Blood* 56:145–158, 1980.

65. Barnard, D. R., and Arthur, M. M. Fibronectin (cold insoluble globulin) in the neonate. *J. Pediatr.* 102:453–455, 1983.

66. Yoder, M. C. et al. Plasma fibronectin in healthy newborn infants: respiratory distress syndrome and perinatal asphyxia. *J. Pediatr.* 102:777–780, 1983.

67. Gerdes, J. S. et al. Decreased plasma fibronectin in neonatal sepsis. *Pediatrics* 72:877–881, 1983.

68. Hill, H. R. et al. Fibronectin deficiency: a correctable defect in the neonate's host defense mechanism (abstr.). *Pediatr. Res.* 17:252A, 1983.

F O U R

Clinical Antecedents

A number of clinical situations place infants at particular risk, irrespective of birth weight or gestation. In some cases these situations are related to prenatal events and in others to postnatal events.

Amniotic Fluid Infection

Among the factors that increase the risk of neonatal infection, infection of amniotic fluid clearly is important.[1-3] The diagnosis, however, may present fewer problems for the pathologist: from a clinical standpoint, amniotic fluid infection or chorioamnionitis is not always easy to ascertain.[4,5] Prolonged rupture of membranes (i.e., longer than 24 hours), however, has been associated with infection and maternal fever is usually an ominous sign. In older studies, the incidence of intrauterine infection seemed to rise rapidly after rupture of membranes, being 10% within 48 hours, 26% by 72 hours, and 40% beyond that time.[6] More recent studies have suggested that a more conservative approach to premature rupture of the membranes may not produce an increasing risk with duration of rupture. In one study of 116 pregnancies between 28 and 36 weeks with ruptured membranes, 9 infants developed neonatal sepsis.[7] The incidence was 1 in 24 (4.2%), 2 in 31 (6.5%), 3 in 27 (11.1%), and 3 in 45 (6.6%) with membranes ruptured less than 24 hours, 24 to 48 hours, 48 to 72 hours, or greater than 72 hours, respectively.[7] (On the other hand, respiratory distress seemed to decrease with progressive duration of ruptured membranes.)

In another study, 329 neonates were evaluated from several high-risk situations with an overall incidence of septicemia of 3%; the incidence was 20% in those infants born to mothers with fever.[8] It has also been suggested that maternal fever is an unreliable prognostic indicator.[9] Salem and Thadepalli noted that although the histologic features of chorioamnionitis may be a fairly common finding, such findings are infrequently associated with clinical sepsis of the newborn.[10]

In addition to these classic associations, an increasing body of evidence supports the idea that either preterm labor or premature rupture of membranes (rupture prior to labor) may be associated with bacterial growth in the amniotic fluid.[6,11] It has been noted that the amniotic fluid of well-nourished women has bacteriostatic properties; therefore, amniotic fluid is usually sterile.[12] For a number of reasons bacteria may traverse the membrane barrier and infect the amniotic fluid, resulting in either preterm labor or premature rupture of the membranes.[11,13,14] In a study from South Africa, 72% (40) of 56 preterm infants came from an infected intrauterine environment.[13] Amniotic fluid infection seems to be more prevalent in women who are poorly nourished or who come from the lower socioeconomic groups.[15] The presence of adequate amounts of zinc in the amniotic fluid may help to suppress bacterial growth, but dietary zinc supplementation does not appear to prevent amniotic fluid infection (see chapter 2).

Ruptured membranes are not a prerequisite of infection:[14] membranes may rupture or premature labor begin as the *result* of infection.[6,11] In order to document the presence of infection it may be necessary to obtain amniotic fluid by amniocentesis[14] or possibly via an intrauterine pressure catheter, which is used for fetal monitoring.[16] Using the latter method, bacterial colony counts in excess of 10^7 colony forming units per milliliter seemed to be associated with clinical illness and increased neonatal risk.[16]

Another method proposed to detect chorioamnionitis is the measurement of C-reactive protein (CRP) levels.[17,18] When first described this seemed to be a very valuable test with no false-positives in 109 patients.[17] In 14 of 20 patients followed serially, CRP levels became elevated at least 12 hours before any other finding. A more recent experience, however, casts some doubt on the value of CRP testing in clinical decisions.[18] On the other hand, the ability to suppress preterm labor with tocolytic agents correlated strongly with negative CRP findings (i.e., tocolysis failed with a positive CRP).[18a]

Although culture of amniotic fluid requires several hours to obtain a result, it may be possible to detect the presence of pathogenic bacteria quite rapidly by using gas-liquid chromatography.[19] Abnormal patterns of organic acids in amniotic fluid can detect infection in approximately 1 hour on as little as 1 ml of amniotic fluid. Lactate seems to be predominant throughout pregnancy, but acetate, succinate, butyrate, and other organic acids may indicate bacterial metabolites.[19] In a study of 16 patients with amniotic fluid infection and 22 noninfected patients, 15 of 16 had an abnormal pattern on gas-liquid chromatography in the infected group, compared with only 1 of 22 in the control group.[19]

Despite the ability to make a clinical diagnosis of chorioamnionitis or amniotic fluid infection, it should be remembered that the frequency of documented early-onset neonatal sepsis under such circumstances is only 3% to 8%.[8,20] Whether or not the more objective measures described in the preceding paragraphs will correlate with a higher percentage of infections is not clear at this time.

Maternal Infection and Colonization

Preterm delivery has been associated with maternal urinary tract infection[21] and results in infants who are more susceptible to neonatal sepsis (see chapter 2). In addition, there is an increased incidence of amniotic fluid infection with urinary tract infection so that these circumstances may conspire to place the neonate at increased risk.[1,2] Despite these associations, a recent study of 487 pregnant women with acute pyelonephritis showed that antepartum infection can be treated with no increase in adverse outcome. With intrapartum infection, pyelonephritis appeared to have initiated labor in some cases.[22]

Another circumstance, fortunately infrequent, is the presence of maternal sepsis, which increases the chance of neonatal sepsis.[1,2,23] Because maternal sepsis is easier to diagnose than urinary tract infection, appropriate therapy can be given to the mother before delivery, and may also treat the baby.

The most likely source of bacteria in amniotic fluid infection is the vaginal flora. Pathogenic bacteria may be acquired by the neonate during vaginal delivery. In particular, much attention has been given to colonization and infection of the neonate with group B streptococci (GBS). Some studies have reported as many as 25% or more of pregnant women are colonized with GBS.[28] In other recent reports as few as 5% to 10% have been colonized.[29-31] Ten to fifty percent of neonatal GBS colonization is believed to be acquired from colonized mothers; however, only 1% to 2% of GBS neonatal sepsis may be caused by colonized mothers.[28-31] It seems likely that enhanced transmission of GBS occurs with the use of intrauterine fetal monitors.[32]

While the incidence of systemic infection with GBS (i.e., sepsis, pneumonia, and meningitis) was approximately 1 to 4 per 1000 live births in the 1970s,[28] neonatal sepsis caused by *Escherichia coli* has remained more constant—approximately 0.5 to 1.0 per 1000 live births—since the introduction of antibiotics.[33] Obviously, it is very common for the neonate to be exposed to coliform organisms because of the anatomic proximity of the colon to the vagina. In a recent study, 8% of women had bacteriuria in pregnancy, and *E. coli* was the most common organism isolated (more frequent than GBS); bacteriuria therefore may be another source of this organism.[34]

Importance of Cervical Cerclage

In patients with a history of preterm labor, it has recently been suggested that a more aggressive approach to using cervical cerclage might be helpful, the rationale being that prevention of cervical dilatation might prevent the interaction of vaginal flora with the fetal membranes by reducing the area of exposure.[11] When cervical cerclage is attempted in the latter part of the second trimester of pregnancy, however, a markedly increased risk of chorioamnionitis seems to be present. In a study of 115 patients, the optimal time suggested to perform cervical cerclage was the 14th to 18th week; later in the second trimester, the incidence of chorioamnionitis was increased 2.6-fold.[24]

Coitus in Late Pregnancy

The possibility that coitus in late pregnancy contributes to chorioamnionitis and preterm delivery has received a good deal of attention in recent years, but there are wide divergences of opinion on the subject.[25-27] Naeye has documented an association between preterm delivery following premature rupture of the membranes when recent coitus occurred in conjunction with chorioamnionitis.[25] The study involved 10,460 pregnancies, and preterm delivery occurred 11 times more frequently when both recent coitus and chorioamnionitis were present than when both were absent.[25] Naeye and Ross have also suggested that the increased likelihood of chorioamnionitis may be the result of semen carrying bacteria through the barrier of cervical mucus.[26]

In contrast to Naeye's view is the study of Mills and colleagues.[27] They studied 10,981 singleton, low-risk pregnancies and found that preterm delivery was no more frequent in those women having coitus than in those abstaining. They also found no increased risk for premature rupture of membranes, low birth weight, or perinatal death at any gestational age.[27]

Neonatal Asphyxia and Jaundice

In addition to the deficiencies in defense mechanisms discussed in chapter 3, infants who are subjected to asphyxia and who require resuscitation appear to be at particular risk for neonatal sepsis and meningitis.[8,35,36] The reasons for this susceptibility are not at all clear, but the clinical observation has been made repeatedly. Of course, many of the infants at particular risk (e.g., preterm, intrauterine growth-retarded) are also more likely to be subjected to asphyxia, so that it is difficult to determine what additional factors are involved, but the hexose-monophosphate shunt may be involved and complement levels are probably lower (see chapter 3).

Jaundiced infants also seem to be more susceptible to sepsis and there is evidence to show that increased levels of unconjugated bilirubin markedly inhibit the hexose-monophosphate-shunt activity of neutrophils.[37] Neonatal sepsis also may predispose the jaundiced infant to kernicterus.[38]

Invasive Procedures and Neonatal Sepsis

Endotracheal Suctioning

Endotracheal suctioning is among the more common procedures performed in the intensive care nursery. Many infants require assisted ventilation and the use of an endotracheal tube. Although it is unclear how frequently suctioning needs to be performed to maintain patency of the tube, it is generally agreed that it should be performed several times a day (usually in association with instillation of saline). This common practice, though presumably necessary, is potentially dangerous because transient bacteremia may follow suctioning.[39] There is an increased incidence of sepsis in infants on assisted ventilation, which may certainly be caused by frequent suctioning.[39,40] Colonization was significantly more frequent in babies intubated for more than 72 hours, and a total of 12 of 54 intubated babies subsequently developed systemic infection, with *E. coli* the causative organism in 5 infants.[40]

Central Venous Catheters

For many years it has been recognized that central venous catheters place infants at particular risk for sepsis. Initially this association was made with umbilical venous catheters,[41,42] which seemed to have a much higher incidence of associated infection than umbilical artery catheters.[43] The reasons for this are uncertain, but the more sluggish circulation on the venous side may be a contributing factor and an observed high incidence of thrombotic phenomena in venous catheters also may act as a nidus of infection.[44,45] Prophylactic antibiotics do not seem to be helpful in either type, and in some instances there is difficulty in distinguishing between contamination and infection.[42,43,46] One study has suggested that semiquantitative cultures may help to differentiate true infection, particularly with *Staphylococcus epidermidis*.[47]

The more recent introduction of central venous catheters—usually inserted into the jugular veins and thence to the superior vena cava—for the purpose of providing nutrition (total parenteral nutrition or hyperalimentation), led to an associated rise in the incidence of sepsis. Whether or not this was because the infants who required this form of treatment were the sickest and therefore the most vulnerable infants is unclear, but recent evidence supports that contention.[48] Clearly this associated risk induced many clinicians to attempt supplemental (or even total) parenteral nutrition using peripheral veins. Because needles do not usually maintain intravenous infusions for longer than 24 hours (frequently less) and can themselves be associated with sepsis,[49] peripheral venous catheters became more popular, but they too may have the attendant risk of sepsis. Newer catheters and techniques may decrease the incidence of infection with central venous catheters.[50]

Peripheral Artery Catheters

Because it is not always possible to insert an umbilical artery catheter and the potential risks are great, many physicians have used peripheral artery (e.g., radial artery) catheters for blood sampling. These too are not without risk.[51,52] In particular, the risk of sepsis is probably higher than with umbilical artery catheters, but may be minimized by limiting the duration of catheterization. When 147 radial artery catheterizations were evaluated, the mean duration was 48 ± 6 hours, 25.4% (28) of 110 catheters cultured grew bacteria, but there was only 1 case of sepsis.[51] One recent report from Australia actually documented a case of sepsis resulting in death as a complication of a radial artery catheter, and also showed that bacterial colonization was significantly more common in cannulas present for more than 7 days.[52]

Surgery

Once again the reasons may be unclear but there appears to be an association between neonatal surgery and sepsis.[53] This association may be the result of manipulation of areas that are heavily colonized by bacteria (such as the intestine), or there may be compromise of immunologic mechanisms in the postsurgical period.

Practical Applications

Despite the difficulty in making a diagnosis of chorioamnionitis, both obstetricians and pediatricians should be aware that the following clinical situations suggest that an infant is at particular risk for neonatal sepsis:

1. Prolonged rupture of membranes (> 24 hr)

2. Premature, particularly preterm, rupture of membranes (i.e., membranes ruptured before labor contractions are established)

3. Preterm labor without adequate explanation; satisfactory explanations would be multiple pregnancy, abruptio placentae, and so on

4. Meconium-stained amniotic fluid without adequate explanation (it is particularly unusual to see meconium-stained amniotic fluid prior to 36 weeks' gestation—especially < 34 weeks' gestation—and this finding has been associated with *Listeria* infection)

5. Maternal fever or other evidence of maternal infection

6. Fetal tachycardia detected on fetal heart rate monitoring

7. Foul-smelling amniotic fluid or malodorous baby

Some personal observations indicate that when a single risk factor is present, investigation of the infant for neonatal sepsis is relatively unrewarding. Only 2 of 150 babies investigated for a single factor suggesting amniotic fluid infection had sepsis. On the other hand, the yield was considerably improved (13 of 126) when more than one risk factor was present, particularly in the presence of signs suggestive of sepsis in the neonate.[54]

Thus, from a practical point of view, it seems that if an infant is investigated for sepsis only on the basis of a single risk factor, antibiotics could be withheld, although a blood culture might be sent and other simple investigations performed.[55] In the very preterm infant (< 1500 or < 32 weeks) or in the presence of neonatal asphyxia or other signs suggesting neonatal infection, it seems prudent to draw blood for culture (as well as obtaining CSF and possibly urine for the same purpose) and to start appropriate antibiotics. If cultures are negative at 48 hours—or possibly 72 hours—the situation can be reassessed in light of other investigations (see chapters 8 and 11).

References

1. Blanc, W. A. Amniotic infection syndrome. *Clin. Obstet. Gynecol.* 2:725–734, 1959.

2. Bernirschke, K., and Clifford, S. H. Intrauterine bacterial infection of the newborn infant. *J. Pediatr.* 54:11–18, 1959.

3. Naeye, R. L., and Peters, E. C. Amniotic fluid infections with intact membranes leading to perinatal death: a prospective study. *Pediatrics* 61:171–177, 1978.

4. Mead, P. B. Management of the patient with premature rupture of the membranes. *Clin. Perinatol.* 7:243–244, 1980.

5. Gibbs, R. S. et al. Quantitative bacteriology of amniotic fluid from women with clinical intra-amniotic infection at term. *J. Infect. Dis.* 145:1–8, 1982.

6. Premature rupture of the membranes (editorial). *Br. Med. J.* 1:1165–1166, 1979.

7. Varner, M. W., and Galask, R. P. Conservative management of premature rupture of the membranes. *Am. J. Obstet. Gynecol.* 140:39–43, 1981.

8. Knudsen, F. U., and Steinrud, J. Septicemia of the newborn, associated with ruptured fetal membranes, discolored amniotic fluid or maternal fever. *Acta Paediatr. Scand.* 65:725–731, 1976.

9. Evaldson, G.; Lagrelius, A.; and Winiarski, J. Premature rupture of the membranes. *Acta Obstet. Gynecol. Scand.* 59:385–393, 1980.

10. Salem, F. A., and Thadepalli, H. Microbial invasion of the placenta, cord and membranes during active labor: a not infrequent finding, usually unassociated with clinical sepsis of the newborn. *Clin. Pediatr.* 18:50–52, 1979.

11. Minkoff, H. Prematurity: infection as an etiologic factor. *Obstet. Gynecol.* 62:137–144, 1983.

12. Appelbaum, P. C. et al. Studies on the growth-inhibiting property of amniotic fluids from two United States population groups. *Am. J. Obstet. Gynecol.* 137:579–582, 1980.

13. Roos, P. J. et al. The bacteriological environment of preterm infants. *S. Afr. Med. J.* 57:347–350, 1980.

14. Bobitt, J. R.; Hayslip, C. C.; and Damato, J. D. Amniotic fluid infection as determined by transabdominal amniocentesis in patients with intact membranes in premature labor. *Am. J. Obstet. Gynecol.* 140:947–952, 1981.

15. Naeye, R. L., and Blanc, W. A. Relation of poverty and race to antenatal infection. *N. Engl. J. Med.* 283:555–560, 1970.

16. Courcel, R. J. et al. Quantitative bacteriological analysis of amniotic fluid. *Biol. Neonate* 42:166–173, 1982.

17. Evans, M. I. et al. C-reactive protein as a predictor of infectious morbidity with premature rupture of membranes. *Am. J. Obstet. Gynecol.* 138:648–652, 1980.

18. Farb, H. F. et al. C-reactive protein with premature rupture of membranes and premature labor. *Obstet. Gynecol.* 62:49–51, 1983.

18a. Handwerker, S. M. et al. Correlation of maternal serum C-reactive protein with outcome of tocolysis. *Obstet. Gynecol.* 63:220–224, 1984.

19. Gravett, M. G. et al. Rapid diagnosis of amniotic fluid infection by gas-liquid chromatography. *N. Engl. J. Med.* 306:725–728, 1982.

20. Yoder, P. R. et al. A prospective, controlled study of maternal and perinatal outcome after intra-amniotic infection at term. *Am. J. Obstet Gynecol.* 145:695–701, 1983.

21. Naeye, R. L. Causes of the excessive rates of perinatal mortality and prematurity in pregnancies complicated by maternal urinary tract infections. *N. Engl. J. Med.* 300:819–823, 1979.

22. Gilstrap, L. C. et al. Renal infection and pregnancy outcome. *Am. J. Obstet. Gynecol.* 141:709–716, 1981.

23. Pass, M. A.; Gray, B. M.; and Dillon, H. C., Jr. Puerperal and perinatal infections with group B streptococci. *Am. J. Obstet. Gynecol.* 143:147–152, 1982.

24. Charles, D., and Edwards, W. R. Infectious complications of cervical cerclage. *Am. J. Obstet. Gynecol.* 141:1065–1071, 1981.

25. Naeye, R. L. Factors that predispose to premature rupture of the fetal membranes. *Obstet. Gynecol.* 60:93–98, 1982.

26. Naeye, R. L., and Ross, S. Coitus and chorioamnionitis: a prospective study. *Early Hum. Dev.* 6(1):91–97, 1982.

27. Mills, J. L.; Harlap, S.; and Harley, E. E. Should coitus late in pregnancy be discouraged? *Lancet* 2:136–138, 1981.

28. Baker, C. J. Group B streptococcal infections in neonates. *Pediatrics in Review* 1:5–15, 1979.

29. Gerard, P. et al. Group B streptococcal colonization of pregnant women and their neonates: epidemiological study and controlled trial of prophylactic treatment of the newborn. *Acta Paediatr. Scand.* 68:819–823, 1979.

30. Lewin, E. B., and Amstey, M. S. Natural history of group B streptococcus colonization and its therapy during pregnancy. *Am. J. Obstet. Gynecol.* 139:512–515, 1981.

31. Anthony, B. F. Carriage of group B streptococci during pregnancy: a puzzler. *J. Infect. Dis.* 145:789–793, 1982.

32. Davis, J. P. et al. Vertical transmission of group B streptococcus: relation to intrauterine fetal monitoring. *J.A.M.A.* 242:42–44, 1979.

33. Freedman, R. M. et al. A half century of neonatal sepsis at Yale: 1928 to 1978. *Am. J. Dis. Child.* 135:140–144, 1981.

34. Wood, E. G., and Dillon, H. C., Jr. A prospective study of group B streptococcal bacteriuria in pregnancy. *Am. J. Obstet. Gynecol.* 140:515–520, 1981.

35. Töllner, U., and Pohlandt, F. Septicemia in the newborn due to gram-negative bacilli: risk factors, clinical symptoms and hematologic changes. *Eur. J. Pediatr.* 123:243–254, 1976.

36. Amiel-Tison, C.; Pilla Grossi, S.; and Henrion, R. Maternal transmission of bacterial infections in 67 newborn infants. *J. Gynecol. Obstet. Biol. Reprod.* (Paris) 9:479–487, 1980.

37. Thong, Y. H., and Rencis, V. Bilirubin inhibits hexose-monophosphate shunt activity of phagocytosing neutrophils. *Acta Paediatr. Scand.* 66:757–759, 1977.

38. Pearlman, M. A. et al. The association of kernicterus with bacterial infection in the newborn. *Pediatrics* 65:26–29, 1980.

39. Storm, W. Transient bacteremia following endotracheal suctioning in ventilated newborns. *Pediatrics* 65:487–490, 1980.

40. Harris, H.; Wirtschafter, D.; and Cassady, G. Endotracheal intubation and its relationship to bacterial colonization and systemic infection of newborn infants. *Pediatrics* 58:816–823, 1976.

41. Krauss, A. N.; Albert, R. F.; and Kannon, M. M. Contamination of umbilical catheters in the newborn infant. *J. Pediatr.* 77:965–969, 1970.

42. Balagtas, R. C. et al. Risk of local and systemic infection associated

with umbilical vein catheterization: a prospective study in 86 newborn patients. *Pediatrics* 48:359–367, 1971.

43. Wesstrom, G., and Finnstrom, O. Umbilical artery catheterization in newborns. II: Infections in relation to catheterization. *Acta Paediatr. Scand.* 68:713–718, 1979.

44. Larroche, J. C. Umbilical catheterization: its complications: anatomical study. *Biol. Neonate* 16:101–116, 1970.

45. Wigger, H. J.; Bransilver, B. R., and Blanc, W. A. Thrombosis due to catheterization in infants and children. *J. Pediatr.* 76:1–11, 1970.

46. Van Vliet, P. K. J., and Gupta, J. M. Prophylactic antibiotics in umbilical artery catheterization in the newborn. *Arch. Dis. Child.* 48:296–300, 1973.

47. Adam, R. D. et al. Semiquantitative cultures and routine tip cultures on umbilical catheters. *J. Pediatr.* 100:123–126, 1982.

48. Placzek, M. M., and Whitelaw, A. Early and late neonatal septicaemia. *Arch. Dis. Child.* 58:728–731, 1983.

49. Harbin, R. L., and Schaffner, W. Septicemia associated with scalp-vein needles. *South Med. J.* 66:638–640, 1973.

50. Loeff, D. S. et al. Insertion of a small central venous catheter in neonates and young infants. *J. Pediatr. Surg.* 17:944–948, 1982.

51. Adams, J. M.; Speer, M. E.; and Rudolph, A. J. Bacterial colonization of radial artery catheters. *Pediatrics* 65:94–97, 1980.

52. Leslie, G. I.; Barr, P. A.; and Pritchard, R. C. Bacterial infection of peripheral artery cannulae in newborn infants. *Aust. Paediatr. J.* 17:283–284, 1981.

53. Eriksson, M. Neonatal septicemia. *Acta Paediatr. Scand.* 72:1–8, 1983.

54. Philip, A. G. S. Neonatal sepsis resulting from possible amniotic fluid infection. *Clin. Pediatr.* 21:210–214, 1982.

55. Philip, A. G. S. Decreased use of antibiotics using a neonatal sepsis screening technique. *J. Pediatr.* 98:795–799, 1981.

F I V E

Clinical Manifestations

The difficulty in making a diagnosis of neonatal sepsis is largely attributable to the wide variety of clinical features that can indicate sepsis at an early stage in the course of the illness.[1-7] The importance of recognizing these clinical manifestations rests with the fact that failure to treat at an early stage is likely to result in high mortality and morbidity.

Many neonates with these clinical features do not prove to have infection. In fact, it is safe to say that most babies who display the assorted features suggesting sepsis, who then have a "sepsis work-up" performed, do not prove to have sepsis. Nevertheless, it is important to consider what these features are, as some of them will have greater significance at different postnatal ages or different gestational ages.

Some clinical features are so suggestive of sepsis, that there is usually little delay in making a diagnosis. With others, there may be many alternative explanations. Some of these will be considered in more detail here.

Early Signs

Lethargy

Finding an objective definition of lethargy that all would agree on is difficult; however, it is generally understood that a "lethargic" baby is

55

one who is difficult to arouse at times when one would expect to be able to arouse the baby. Thus, this definition does not include the term baby who has just been fed, where the greatest difficulty may be encountered in rousing the baby from sleep. Similarly, preterm infants with respiratory distress syndrome may not be particularly interested in their environment. The infant born following prolonged magnesium sulfate administration or following prolapse of the umbilical cord may be very difficult to arouse and considered lethargic, but the diagnosis of sepsis would not immediately be entertained.

Low Apgar Scores

In the absence of maternal administration of general anaesthetic or analgesic and without evidence of fetal asphyxia, a baby may be "depressed" at birth (shown by a low Apgar score) on the basis of sepsis. Although this is really an extension of lethargy, it is the earliest observable neonatal manifestation of systemic infection.

Poor Feeding

The difficulty in defining lethargy extends to poor feeding. What is usually implied is that a baby who was formerly taking nipple feedings quite vigorously, now does so reluctantly or not at all. Consequently, the preterm infant of gestational age less than 32 weeks is difficult to include in this category, because adequate sucking is not present until about 32 weeks' gestation. "Difficulty with feeding" may extend to infants who are gavage, or tube fed, as increasing gastric residuals or poor gastric emptying can suggest an underlying infectious problem.

Abdominal Distention

It is a little easier to be objective about abdominal distention, as abdominal circumference (girth) can be measured sequentially. Even sequential measurement is not entirely reliable, because a vigorous infant who is swallowing a lot of air may have increased abdominal circumference because of air-filled loops of bowel. Under these circumstances the abdomen usually remains soft. An abdomen that appears somewhat tense (particularly if it is shiny) would be more indicative of sepsis. Particularly in the baby weighing less than 1500 g the possibility of necrotizing enterocolitis (NEC) also exists, but, as bacterial infection is probably also implicated in NEC, the mangement is usually very similar. It may be important to remember that abdominal distention in the first 24 to 48 hours postdelivery, particularly in the absence of stool, is more likely to be caused by a mid- or lower intestinal obstruction.

Temperature Instability

Temperature instability can be defined more or less exactly by setting limits for fever or hypothermia. Contrary to the situation in older children, fever in the neonate in response to bacterial infection is comparatively unusual. This is particularly true in preterm infants in whom low body temperature (hypothermia) is more likely to occur. No abnormality of body temperature is probably more common than either hypothermia or fever. In addition, fluctuating body temperature—though still within the limits set as normal—may require investigation, and difficulties in maintaining temperature in babies attached to temperature servocontrol devices should also cause concern.

In the first few hours after delivery (approximately the first 4 hours), abnormal temperatures may be more difficult to assess. Fever in the neonate may be the result of maternal fever, as the fetal temperature usually is approximately 0.5° C above the mother's temperature.[8] Hypothermia, particularly in the small baby, may be the result of cooling in the delivery room, as greater heat loss tends to occur in that setting than subsequently. Hypothermia itself may predispose to infection, especially after 3 days of age.[9]

One further observation is worthy of note. It was observed many years ago that babies with fever caused by increased environmental temperature usually felt warm all over, while babies with sepsis had an elevated core temperature (i.e., the trunk felt warm), but cooling of the extremities. This "tummy-toe" differential was described by Oliver[10] and Segal,[11] and recently has been more accurately documented by Pomerance and colleagues using a skin thermistor and an abdomen-leg difference.[12] Their preliminary experience suggests that differences greater than 3° F—particularly above 5° F—are indicative of bacterial infection (sepsis).

As mentioned earlier, fever after the first 24 hours is a relatively uncommon manifestation in the neonatal period. Another recent study showed that when fever *was* present, it was a highly sensitive indicator of sepsis in term infants.[13] On the other hand, its positive predictive value for sepsis was only 10% (i.e., 10 of 100 febrile term newborns had culture-proved sepsis). The predictive value increased after the first 48 hours.[13] Similarly, a very high incidence of infection was noted when infants presented with hypothermia (t° < 35° C) after 72 hours of age.[9] Of 44 infected infants among 67 with hypothermia between 4 and 28 days of age, 12 had sepsis and 7 had meningitis.[9]

Fever after the immediate neonatal period may be even less predictive of neonatal sepsis, but needs careful evaluation. In a study of 175 infants less than 8 weeks of age presenting with fever (t° > 38° C) in an emergency room, culture-positive bacterial infections occurred in 11 (6.3%) and 6 (3.4%) had bacteremia.[14]

Apnea

There is perhaps no other sign of sepsis with a greater number of differential diagnoses than apnea. The many different etiologies of apnea include a large number of disorders of the lung, acidosis, metabolic disorders (e.g., hypoglycemia), intracranial hemorrhage, and many other disorders that contribute to neonatal seizures (apnea may be a "seizure equivalent"), not to mention "apnea of prematurity."

Nevertheless, apnea frequently initiates a search for infection, whether for sepsis or meningitis, and one would certainly hesitate to make a diagnosis of "apnea of prematurity" without first ruling out sepsis or meningitis. In some series apnea has been described as a frequently associated feature of neonatal sepsis. This may be particularly true of early-onset group B streptococcal (GBS) sepsis and pneumonia, especially in the first 24 hours after delivery.[15,16] In the absence of lung disease, apnea occurring after the first week of extrauterine life would certainly raise the possibility of meningitis.

Cyanotic Episodes

In much the same way that many other disorders may produce apnea, many disorders may produce cyanotic episodes, or "dusky spells." For instance, "potentially cyanotic" congenital heart disease, hyperviscosity (high hematocrit) syndrome, and lung disorders quickly come to mind. Even if cyanotic episodes are rather nonspecific, if some of the other conditions briefly alluded to do not seem to be present, sepsis, meningitis, or both should be seriously considered.

Respiratory Distress

Although apnea and cyanotic episodes arguably constitute respiratory distress, respiratory distress usually implies dyspnea or labored breathing, with the frequent association of grunting and retractions of the intercostal spaces (and sternum). The primary concern is to differentiate pneumonia from respiratory distress syndrome (RDS); however, pneumonia frequently is associated with sepsis. For instance, in a study from Australia of 11 patients with early-onset pneumonia, 9 had positive blood cultures.[16] In the term infant (or the infant born close to term), the chances that dyspnea is the result of RDS are considerably less than in the preterm infant, so that the probability of pneumonia and sepsis is increased accordingly, especially if evidence of lung maturity can be demonstrated.[17] In the preterm infant, it can be almost impossible on clinical and radiographic grounds to distinguish between the two. Although the greatest number of studies have been concerned with distinguishing RDS from GBS pneumonia,[15,18-22] other organisms including pneumococcus, *Haemophilus influenzae*, and *Escherichia coli*, can produce an almost identical picture.[23-25] The difficulty in differentiating the radiographic picture probably results from the pathologic association of hyaline membranes (with engulfed organisms) with some cases of pneumonia[24-26] and the presence in RDS of hyaline membranes as the principal pathologic abnormality; in fact, hyaline membrane disease is the synonym for RDS.

Irritability

Just as lethargy is not easy to define, it is also difficult to accurately define irritability. Irritability is usually considered to be present when an infant seems more restless than usual for a given gestational age, when any stimulus seems to provoke tremulousness or increased activity, or when a baby cries intermittently for no apparent reason.

Once again, a number of disorders of the central nervous system can produce this clinical picture, particularly hypoxic-ischemic encephalopathy and intracranial hemorrhage in its various forms. Meningitis, however, must also be seriously considered and appropriate investigations carried out to determine whether or not it is present. Irritability occurring in the first 3 days after delivery is most likely to be due to hypoxic-ischemic encephalopathy or intracranial hemorrhage. After 3 days, particularly if an infant becomes irritable for the first time, meningitis becomes increasingly more likely as each day passes. Although most cases of meningitis present after the seventh day of age, approximately 30% occur during the first week.[4]

Jaundice

As with apnea and cyanotic episodes, there are multiple etiologies of neonatal jaundice. The distinction between the various causes is largely determined by the age at presentation, but jaundice at any age in the neonatal period can be caused by sepsis. In certain circumstances jaundice caused by sepsis would be unusual. In the first 24 hours after birth blood group incompatibility remains the most likely explanation for jaundice. Because physiologic jaundice is so common 3 and 4 days' postdelivery, jaundice caused by sepsis is unlikely unless some other sign of sepsis is also present.

Although the increased bilirubin in neonatal sepsis is usually predominantly in the unconjugated, or indirect, fraction, it is not uncommon to see some elevation of the conjugated, or direct, fraction. This seems to be particularly true with coliform organisms, especially in association with urinary tract infection, and is presumably caused by mild hepatocellular swelling.[27-29] If there is marked hepatic involvement, quite high levels of conjugated bilirubin may be seen, but this is uncommon.[29]

A further complicating factor (discussed in chapter 3) is that infants who are jaundiced (for whatever reason) may be particularly susceptible to infection. Thus, the possibility of neonatal sepsis must be considered in any jaundiced infant who displays any other clinical feature suggestive of sepsis.

Hepatosplenomegaly

As mentioned earlier, some degree of hepatocellular swelling is not uncommon in association with neonatal sepsis. Although this feature was noted frequently in earlier reports[3,30] and may occur relatively early, it is an unusual reason for initiating a sepsis work-up, particularly as an isolated feature. More typically, when evaluating an infant with other signs of sepsis, some enlargement of the liver is found and it is not unusual to find some degree of splenic enlargement (i.e., the spleen tip becomes easily palpable in the flank).

Diarrhea and Vomiting

Although more commonly seen in somewhat older infants, systemic infection, including sepsis and meningitis, can be associated with the signs of gastroenteritis without the presence of intestinal involvement. This is sometimes referred to as parenteral vomiting and diarrhea, and may be secondary to the release of endotoxin or endotoxinlike substances.

Pustules and Other Skin Eruptions

Pustules are usually staphylococcal in origin and may be seen around the umbilicus, in the groin, and in other skin folds (e.g., neck and axilla). They are more typically seen later in the neonatal period (i.e., after the first week). By themselves, pustules do not indicate sepsis, but they act as a warning sign. If there is any concern that an infant is not behaving normally at the same time that pustules are present, sepsis should be given serious consideration.[31]

Bullae may be more ominous markers of staphylococcal infection and other skin lesions may also suggest that sepsis should be sought. For example, *Pseudomonas* infection may produce violaceous skin lesions that develop necrotic centers, which suggest that the infection is blood-borne.[30,32]

Although petechiae and purpura can be indications of thrombocytopenia and may also suggest a diagnosis of sepsis, they may be comparatively late features.

The major clinical features suggesting neonatal sepsis, meningitis, or both have been evaluated by Wientzen and McCracken in a literature review.[33] The frequency of each presenting feature is outlined in table 5.1, but should be interpreted with caution; some of the features considered common may be quite nonspecific and relate to the era in which the data were gathered (see also Appendix tables 1–3).

Late or Ominous Signs

Pallor

Any cause of metabolic acidosis may result in peripheral vascoconstriction with resultant pallor. Although metabolic acidosis is not usually present in the early stages of neonatal sepsis, it should always raise the possibility of sepsis in the absence of other more obvious etiologies (e.g., blood loss). Peripheral vasoconstriction or pallor or both may occur as the result of release of endotoxin or endotoxinlike substances from pathogenic bacteria. This sign suggests that there is little time to lose in initiating treatment and other possible reasons for pallor should be only briefly investigated before performing cultures and starting antibiotics. In a retrospective analysis of 83 infants with septicemia, Töllner reported that abnormal skin color, impaired capillary filling time,

Table 5.1.
Frequency of Clinical Manifestations Seen in Neonatal Sepsis and Meningitis

	No. of cases/total cases	Incidence (%)
Fever	137/353	39
Jaundice	110/369	30
Hepatomegaly	96/318	30
Poor feeding	94/323	29
Respiratory distress	100/348	29
Apnea	27/117	23
Cyanotic episodes	57/248	23
Abdominal distention	51/248	21
Vomiting	47/223	21
Rash	28/151	19
Irritability	23/135	17
Diarrhea	44/294	15
Lethargy	53/369	14
Hypothermia	17/117	14

Modified from R. L. Wientzen, Jr., and G. H. McCracken, Jr. Pathogenesis and management of neonatal sepsis and meningitis. *Curr. Probl. Pediatr.* 8(2):1–61, 1977.

and metabolic acidosis were seen in 78%, 46%, and 24%, respectively, at the onset of the illness and in 95%, 95%, and 66%, respectively, at the peak of the disease.[7]

Shock

Markedly compromised peripheral perfusion may indicate systemic hypotension rather than peripheral vasoconstriction. The most reliable way to document this is with blood pressure measurements, either direct (i.e., intra-arterial) or indirect (using the newer noninvasive oscillometric devices). The presence of shock is one stage worse than pallor, and may be accompanied by mottling or blotchiness of the skin (i.e., areas of blotchy erythema alternating with pallor), which is a late sign of sepsis.[5]

Sclerema

The finding of sclerema is usually an ominous sign in any infant and is characterized by a firmness of the subcutaneous tissues that is similar to hard wax (tallowlike) and may even become almost like wood ("woody feel"). Sclerema is almost certainly secondary to decreased peripheral perfusion, as noted earlier. The decreased perfusion results in cooling of the tissues at the periphery—particularly the arms and legs—and a physical alteration in the subcutaneous fat. When this sign is present, extreme measures, such as exchange transfusion (see chapter 11), have been instituted.[34,35]

Petechiae and Purpura

Although thrombocytopenia is considered by some to be a common accompaniment of neonatal sepsis, most investigators in North America consider this to be a late manifestation (see also chapter 9). Because the most frequent manifestations of thrombocytopenia are petechiae and purpura, it is reasonable to assume that they will be present late in the course of neonatal sepsis. It is possible, however, to have petechiae without obvious thrombocytopenia, but the mechanism is obscure—possibly a direct effect of endotoxin.

Convulsions

Irritability was noted earlier to be a possible manifestation of neonatal sepsis and particularly meningitis. A more extreme feature of irritability is the occurrence of a seizure, or convulsion. Seizures do not usually occur in the early stages of meningitis; therefore, the presence of seizure activity is an ominous sign. As with many other signs of sepsis and meningitis, there are several different reasons for neonatal seizures[36]; however, particularly after the first 3 or 4 days, the possibility of meningitis should occur and a lumbar puncture (spinal tap) is mandatory.

Bulging Fontanelle and Nuchal Rigidity

It is unusual for the neonate to exhibit the clinical manifestations that are characteristic of meningitis in older children, however, they are seen from time to time.[37] Particularly in infants who remain in hospital, the signs of bulging fontanelle and nuchal rigidity are considered late signs of meningitis; however, they are seen occasionally in infants who have been at home for a while, in whom the diagnosis of meningitis has been delayed. An additional reason for the rarity of these findings is that the neonatal skull is compliant and can accommodate some increase in pressure by spreading the sutures. This is truer of the preterm than the term infant and is exemplified by a study published in 1961.[38] In 16 preterm infants, none presented early with either a bulging fontanelle or nuchal rigidity, but nuchal rigidity later developed in 1 infant. In 23 term infants, again there were none with these findings initially, but bulging fontanelles later developed in 13 infants and 6 exhibited nuchal rigidity.[38]

References

1. Gotoff, S. P., and Behrman, R. E. Neonatal septicemia. *J. Pediatr.* 76:142–153, 1970.

2. Davies, P. A. Bacterial infection in the fetus and newborn. *Arch. Dis. Child.* 46:1–27, 1971.

3. Quie, P. G. Neonatal septicemia. *Antibiot. Chemother.* 21:128–134, 1976.

4. Daum, R. S., and Smith, A. L. Bacterial sepsis in the newborn. *Clin. Obstet. Gynecol.* 22:385–408, 1979.

5. Neonatal bacteraemia: diagnosis and management (editorial). *Br. Med. J.* 2:1385–1386, 1979.

6. Siegel, J. D., and McCracken, G. H., Jr. Sepsis neonatorum. *N. Engl. J. Med.* 304:642–647, 1981.

7. Töllner, U. Early diagnosis of septicemia in the newborn: clinical studies and sepsis score. *Eur. J. Pediatr.* 138:331–337, 1982.

8. Adamsons, K., Jr. The role of thermal factors in fetal and neonatal life. *Pediatr. Clin. North Am.* 13:599–619, 1966.

9. Sahib El-Radhi, A. et al. Sepsis and hypothermia in the newborn infant: value of gastric aspirate examination. *J. Pediatr.* 103:300–302, 1983.

10. Oliver, T. K., Jr. Temperature regulation and heat production in the newborn. *Pediatr. Clin. North Am.* 12:765–778, 1965.

11. Segal, S. Neonatal intensive care: a prediction of continuing development. *Pediatr. Clin. North Am.* 13:1149–1193, 1966.

12. Pomerance, J. J.; Brand, R. J.; and Meredith, J. L. Differentiating environmental from disease-related fevers in the term newborn. *Pediatrics* 67:485–488, 1981.

13. Voora, S. et al. Fever in full-term newborns in the first four days of life. *Pediatrics* 69:40–44, 1982.

14. Crain, E. F., and Shelov, S. P. Febrile infants: predictors of bacteremia. *J. Pediatr.* 101:686–689, 1982.

15. Ablow, R. C. et al. A comparison of early-onset group B streptococcal neonatal infection and the respiratory distress syndrome of the newborn. *N. Engl. J. Med.* 294:65–70, 1976.

16. Leslie, G. I.; Scurr, R. D.; and Barr, P. A. Early-onset bacterial pneumonia: a comparison with severe hyaline membrane disease. *Aust. Pediatr. J.* 17:202–206, 1981.

17. Jacob, J.; Edwards, D.; and Gluck, L. Early-onset sepsis and pneumonia observed as respiratory distress syndrome: assessment of lung maturity. *Am. J. Dis. Child.* 134:766–768, 1980.

18. Katzenstein, A.; Davis, C.; and Braude, A. Pulmonary changes in neonatal sepsis due to group B beta-hemolytic streptococcus: relation to hyaline membrane disease. *J. Infect. Dis.* 133:430–435, 1976.

19. Leonidas, J. C. et al. Radiographic findings in early onset neonatal group B streptococcal septicemia. *Pediatrics* 59:1006–1011, 1977.

20. Lilien, L. D.; Harris, V. J.; and Pildes, R. S. Significance of radiographic findings in early-onset group B streptococcal infection. *Pediatrics* 60:360–363, 1977.

21. Menke, J. A.; Giacoia, G. P.; and Jockin, H. Group B beta-hemolytic streptococcal sepsis and the idiopathic respiratory distress syndrome: a comparison. *J. Pediatr.* 94:467–471, 1979.

22. Modanlou, H. D.; Bosu, S. K.; and Weller, M. H. Early onset group B streptococcus neonatal septicemia and respiratory distress syndrome: characteristic features of assisted ventilation in the first 24 hours of life. *Crit. Care Med.* 8:716–720, 1980.

23. Bortolussi, R.; Thompson, T. R.; and Ferrieri, P. Early onset pneumococcal sepsis in newborn infants. *Pediatrics* 60:352–355, 1977.

24. Jeffery, H. et al. Early neonatal bacteraemia: comparison of group B streptococcal, other gram-positive and gram-negative infections. *Arch. Dis. Child.* 52:683–686, 1977.

25. Lilien, L. D. et al. Early onset *Hemophilus* sepsis in newborn infants: clinical, roentgenographic and pathologic features. *Pediatrics* 62:299–303, 1978.

26. Craig, J. M. Group B beta hemolytic streptococcal sepsis in the newborn. *Perspect. Pediatr. Pathol.* 6:139–151, 1981.

27. Rooney, J. C.; Hill, D. J.; and Danks, D. M. Jaundice associated with bacterial infection in the newborn. *Am. J. Dis. Child.* 122:39–43, 1971.

28. Seeler, R. A. Urosepsis with jaundice due to hemolytic *Escherichia coli* (letter). *Am. J. Dis. Child.* 126:414, 1973.

29. Watkins, J. B.; Sunaryo, F. P.; and Berezin, S. H. Hepatic manifestations of congenital and perinatal disease. *Clin. Perinatol.* 8:467–480, 1981.

30. Nyhan, W. L., and Fousek, M. D. Septicemia of the newborn. *Pediatrics* 22:268–278, 1958.

31. Holzman, R. S.; Florman, A. L.; and Lyman, M. Gentamicin resistant and sensitive strains of *S. aureus*. Factors affecting colonization and virulence for infants in a special care nursery. *Am. J. Epidemiol.* 112:352–361, 1980.

32. Reed, R. K. et al. Peripheral nodular lesions in *Pseudomonas* sepsis: the importance of incision and drainage. *J. Pediatr.* 88:977–979, 1976.

33. Wientzen, R. L., Jr., and McCracken, G. H., Jr. Pathogenesis and management of neonatal sepsis and meningitis. *Curr. Probl. Pediatr.* 8(2):1–61, 1977.

34. Xanthou, M. et al. Exchange transfusion in severe neonatal infection with sclerema. *Arch. Dis. Child.* 50:901–902, 1975.

35. Vain, N. E. et al. Role of exchange transfusion in the treatment of severe septicemia. *Pediatrics* 66:693–697, 1980.

36. Volpe, J. J. *Neurology of the newborn.* Philadelphia: W. B. Saunders Co., 1981, pp. 111–137 and 536–571.

37. Kairam, R., and DeVivo, D. C. Neurologic manifestations of congenital infection. *Clin. Perinatol.* 8:445–465, 1981.

38. Groover, R. V.; Sutherland, J. M.; and Landing, B. H. Purulent meningitis of newborn infants: eleven year experience with the antibiotic era. *N. Engl. J. Med.* 264:1115–1121, 1961.

S I X

Distant Effects

Several problems associated with neonatal sepsis are not immediately apparent. These problems present in such a way that, unless one is attuned to them, their association with sepsis may be easily overlooked. Although it is probable that all of these clinical difficulties can be thought of as secondary to the primary problem of sepsis, I prefer to call them "distant effects" because they are apparently far removed from the usual presenting features of sepsis.

Cholestasis

As chapter 5 detailed, jaundice is often a presenting feature of neonatal sepsis, but it may be more or less ominous depending on the age of the neonate. Particularly when jaundice presents late in the neonatal period, there is a tendency to think of it as caused by increased hemolysis of red blood cells secondary to the infection. No good evidence, however, supports this concept.[1] Hepatocellular damage is another frequent explanation. Although this explanation seems to be true if one considers periportal infiltration and intrahepatic cholestasis to be evidence of "damage," there is no apparent parenchymal damage (i.e., necrosis). Hepatocellular swelling is a better way to express this concept: electron microscopic studies have shown marked dilatation of microvilli on liver biopsy.[1,2]

 Intrahepatic cholestasis seems to occur much more commonly in association with *Escherichia coli,* especially when there is concomitant urinary tract infection.[1,3] Male neonates apparently are more frequently affected than females.[1,3] In one study of urinary tract infection, the male preponderance was 5 to 1.[4] Evidence points toward the direct effect of endotoxin (released by the *E. coli*) on the hepatocyte.[1,5] For unexplained reasons the neonate seems to have an exaggerated response to the endotoxin, with a giant cell response not seen in adult animals.[6,7] The end result seems to be a great tendency to produce hepatomegaly and to have an associated increase in the fraction of conjugated bilirubin, which may be as high as 10mg/dl.[1]

Although sepsis usually is implicated in the production of cholestasis, recent evidence indicates that sepsis may be more likely in the presence of cholestasis. This was noted in a series of babies who had hyperalimentation-induced cholestasis.[8]

Kernicterus

Considerable controversy exists about the likelihood of developing kernicterus in the presence of comparatively low levels of bilirubin in the preterm infant.[9] Despite little supporting evidence, a standard approach to the preterm infant was to consider exchange transfusion at bilirubin levels that were equated with birth weight (e.g., > 10 mg/dl at 1 kg, > 9 mg/dl at 900 g, and so on). This approach was lent credence by its publication in the handbook of the American Academy of Pediatrics Committee on Fetus and Newborn.[10]

The exact reasons that kernicterus develops in the neonate remain somewhat elusive. Recent evidence points to the "leakage" of bilirubin into the brain following asphyxia; there is also evidence to indicate that acidosis diminishes the binding of bilirubin to albumin.[12] One of the persistent associated reasons for developing kernicterus is neonatal sepsis.[13] The mechanism of this association is not certain, but acidosis is a frequently observed finding in neonatal sepsis. Whether or not endotoxin is also implicated remains speculative.

Persistent Pulmonary Hypertension

The lungs of the fetus are not aerated and there is little advantage in having good blood flow to the lungs. This situation results in increased pulmonary vascular resistance, with pulmonary artery pressure higher than in the systemic arteries and a resultant right to left shunt. This is the normal fetal circulation, and when it persists after delivery, it has been referred to as *persistent fetal circulation*. Because the placenta is no longer in the circuit, *persistent transitional circulation* is a more correct term. More recently the term *persistent pulmonary hypertension* (PPH) has been used to describe this persistence of intrauterine elevated pulmonary artery pressure.

The reasons for PPH are many, but can be broadly categorized as primary and secondary. The usual antecedent of primary PPH is asphyxia and among the many reasons for secondary PPH is group B streptococcal (GBS) sepsis. The exact mechanism again is not completely elucidated, but it seems to be the result of endotoxinlike effects associated with GBS infection.[14,15] There are two possible ways of producing right to left shunting. In addition to having a truly elevated pulmonary artery pressure, it can also be the result of decreased systemic artery pressure (i.e., hypotension or shock) with a relatively normal pulmonary artery pressure. It might be assumed that GBS sepsis would produce PPH by causing shock, but there is also evidence to support a direct effect on pulmonary arterioles.[16]

How many other kinds of infection can produce a similar picture is not known, but the author recently saw an infant with apparent PPH associated with *Haemophilus influenzae* sepsis.[17] There is also experimental animal evidence to indicate that *Staphylococcus aureus,* pneumococcus, and other organisms can produce similar effects.[18,19]

Diaphragmatic Hernia

Among the list of problems associated with GBS infection, one of the most intriguing—and baffling—is the occurrence of right-sided diaphragmatic hernia, which *seems* to be acquired.[20–23] The majority of cases (>80%) of congenital diaphragmatic hernia are reported to be on the left side, but there is always the question whether the liver provides some protection against herniation through a right-sided diaphragmatic defect.

In any event, the association of right-sided diaphragmatic hernia and GBS sepsis was first made in 1978 and has been reported from several different centers since that time. Because there was frequently an associated GBS pneumonia, it has been suggested that the altered pulmonary dynamics may have contributed to herniation through an existing defect. In other cases, however, the pulmonary problem seemed to resolve itself many days before the appearance of the hernia. This observation raises the possibility that GBS infection may selectively weaken the diaphragm on the right side, as no cases have yet been reported on the left. In the "typical" case, there is an interval of 7 to 14 days between the initiation of treatment for GBS sepsis or pneumonia or both and the discovery of a right-sided diaphragmatic hernia.

One other intriguing fact should be mentioned. Although osteomyelitis of the neonate is relatively uncommon, the humerus as well as the maxilla frequently seems to be involved.[24] Commenting on a study of GBS osteomyelitis, Baker remarked that, in contrast to osteomyelitis from other agents, the humerus was almost always affected on the right side.[25]

Other Distant Effects

Transient Hypothyroidism

There are a number of reasons for the development of transient hypothyroidism in neonates. The most frequently associated reasons are prematurity and sick infants who require intensive care. Another frequent association in preterm and sick infants is transient hypothyroxinemia.[26] The distinction between hypothyroxinemia and hypothyroidism is that although the T_4 levels are decreased in both, thyroid-stimulating hormone (TSH) levels are elevated only in hypothyroidism.

In a series from Germany, 60 neonates admitted to an intensive care nursery were evaluated for thyroid function. Seven showed transient hypothyroidism, and of these neonates, four had sepsis.[27] All were less than 37 weeks' gestation and weighed less than 2200 g. The T_4 level was less than 2 μg/dl (3 were <1 μg/dl) and the TSH level was greatly elevated (3 of 4 were >100 μU/ml). The associated organisms were *Klebsiella* and *Pseudomonas*. Although it was not clear whether hypothyroidism was the result of decreased output or increased utilization, the former is more likely.

Hypoglycemia and Hyperglycemia

Hypoglycemia usually is mentioned as an associated finding with neonatal sepsis,[28] but to my knowledge no systematic studies have been performed to determine how frequently it is seen. In the study by Yeung hypoglycemia was associated with gram-negative infection.[29] Subsequent studies have shown an increased disappearance rate of glucose in neonates with infection, but this does not appear to be caused by hyperinsulinism.[30,31] In the study by Leake and colleagues glucose disappearance rates were about three times those of controls in the acute septic period and about twice the control values in the convalescent period.[31] Gram-negative, gram-positive, and viral infections were all associated with this finding, which persisted for 5 to 15 days after treatment was begun.[31] The reason for this rapid glucose disposal remains unclear. Although fever could produce a hypermetabolic state, this is not a prominent feature of neonatal sepsis. Animal evidence points toward increased glucose utilization in the presence of endotoxin.[32]

In addition to *hypo*glycemia, disordered carbohydrate metabolism with *hyper*glycemia has been noted.[33] The presumed mechanism in this case is that the "stress" associated with infection is accompanied by catecholamine and corticosteroid release; these hormones may yield glucose from glycogen stores, with resultant elevation of blood glucose levels.

Hyponatremia

Hyponatremia is most likely to be associated with neonatal meningitis, although it has been noted as a complication of severe septicemia.[28] Because the signs of hyponatremia may be the signs of sepsis, hyponatremia can be overlooked unless serum electrolyte determinations are routinely performed. Hyponatremia is most likely to occur in association with decreased urine output and concentrated urine, when it is part of the syndrome of inappropriate antidiuretic hormone (SIADH). Associated with several disorders of the neonate, SIADH has been linked particularly to asphyxia and neonatal meningitis.[34] Because of this, it may be advisable to limit the fluid intake of meningitic patients. Neonatal pneumonia has also been associated with SIADH.[35]

Cardiovascular Effects

As mentioned earlier, sepsis can cause hypotension (and shock), presumably secondary to endotoxin released. It has also been suggested that the severity of the illness alone can result in cardiac decompensation, with resultant congestive heart failure.[36] This decompensation can also result in decreased cardiac output and poor peripheral perfusion. In addition, intravascular microthrombi (disseminated intravascular coagulation, DIC) may occur as a direct result of the infecting organisms. Corrigan showed that in infants with sepsis who had thrombocytopenia, 11 of 28 had DIC.[37] Zipursky and Jaber, however, believe that DIC is infrequently a direct consequence of infection, but that intravascular coagulation may occur because of cardiac arrest or profound cardiovascular shock.[38] When DIC is present, hemorrhage is more likely. Prolonged bleeding from heelstick blood sampling sites may be the first indication of this phenomenon.

Adrenal Insufficiency

In all cases of meningitis in infancy and childhood, bleeding—hemorrhage—into the adrenal gland is possible. In the past, bleeding was thought to account for poor perfusion and shock as a result of adrenal insufficiency; however, evidence shows that the adrenal is capable of responding to the stress of meningitis, even in the presence of hemorrhage. Thus, although one would hesitate to say that adrenal insufficiency could not occur in neonatal sepsis and meningitis, there is no evidence that adrenal insufficiency does occur.[36]

Associated Focal Infections

A large number of focal infections presumably follow bacteremia that are not necessarily associated with the usual clinical signs of sepsis. Nevertheless, some of these may undoubtedly be associated with sepsis and one should be mindful of them. Neonatal evaluation following a diagnosis of sepsis requires observation for peritonitis,[39] osteomyelitis,[40] hepatic abscess,[41] septic arthritis, and infected cephalhematoma,[42] among others.

Hydrops (mucocele) of the gallbladder

A rather unusual association with neonatal sepsis is the presence of marked enlargement of the gallbladder.[43] Though infrequently reported, it has been associated with group B streptococcal infection and is readily diagnosed with ultrasound. The author recently saw a case in a preterm infant with sepsis due to *Hemophilus influenzae*.

References

1. Watkins, J. B.; Sunaryo, F. P.; and Berezin, S. H. Hepatic manifestations of congenital and perinatal disease. *Clin. Perinatol.* 8:467–480, 1981.

2. Borges, M. A. G.; DeBrito, T.; and Borges, J. M. G. Hepatic manifestations in bacterial infection of infants and children. Clinical features, biochemical data and morphological hepatic changes (histological and ultrastructural). *Acta Hepatol. Gastroenterol.* 19:328, 1972.

3. Kenny, J. F. et al. An outbreak of urinary tract infections and septicemia due to *Escherichia coli* in male infants. *J. Pediatr.* 68:530–541, 1966.

4. Maherzi, M.; Guignard, J. P.; and Torrado, A. Urinary tract infection in high-risk newborn infants. *Pediatrics* 62:521–523, 1978.

5. Zimmerman, H. J. et al. Jaundice due to bacterial infection. *Gastroenterology* 77:362–374, 1979.

6. Nolan, J. P. The role of endotoxin in liver injury. *Gastroenterology* 69:1346–1356, 1975.

7. Utili, R.; Abernathy, C. O.; and Zimmerman, H. J. Cholestatic effects of *Escherichia coli* endotoxin on the isolated perfused rat liver. *Gastroenterology* 70:248–253, 1976.

8. Pereira, G. R. et al. Hyperalimentation-induced cholestasis: increased incidence and severity in premature infants. *Am. J. Dis. Child.* 135:842–845, 1981.

9. Lucey, J. F. Bilirubin and brain damage: a real mess. *Pediatrics* 69:381–382, 1982.

10. Committee on Fetus and Newborn. *Hospital care of newborn infants,* 6th edition. Evanston, Ill.: American Academy of Pediatrics, 1977, p. 95.

11. Levine, R. L.; Fredericks, W. R.; and Rapoport, S. I. Entry of bilirubin into the brain due to opening of the blood-brain barrier. *Pediatrics* 69:255–259, 1982.

12. Cashore, W. J., and Stern, L. Neonatal hyperbilirubinemia. *Pediatr. Clin. North Am.* 29:1191–1203, 1982.

13. Pearlman, M. A. et al. Association of kernicterus with bacterial infection in the newborn. *Pediatrics* 65:26–29, 1980.

14. Shankaran, S.; Farooki, Z. Q.; and Desai, R. β-Hemolytic streptococcal infection appearing as persistent fetal circulation. *Am. J. Dis. Child.* 136:725–727, 1982.

15. Rojas, J. et al. Studies on group B streptococcus: effects on pulmonary hemodynamics and vascular permeability. *Pediatr. Res.* 15:899–904, 1981.

16. Cartwright, D. et al. Endotoxin produces acute pulmonary hypertension and thromboxane elevation in the newborn lamb (abstr.). *Pediatr. Res.* 17:306A, 1983.

17. Hageman, J. R.; Adams, M. A.; and Gardner, T. H. Persistent pulmonary hypertension of the newborn with early onset neonatal infection (abstr.). *Pediatr. Res.* 17:315A, 1983.

18. Shoemaker, S. A. et al. *Staphylococcus aureus* induced platelet aggregation produces acute pulmonary hypertension in isolated perfused rabbit lungs (abstr.). *Am. Rev. Respir. Dis.* 125(Suppl.):97, 1982.

19. Chick, T. W. Pulmonary vascular response to intravascular pneumococcal challenge in dogs (abstr.). *Am. Rev. Respir. Dis.* 125(Suppl.):275, 1982.

20. McCarten, K. M. et al. Delayed onset of right diaphragmatic hernia associated with group B streptococcal infection in the newborn (abstr.). *A. J. R.* 133:435, 1979.

21. Graviss, E. R. et al. Peritoneography: diagnosis of delayed-onset right-sided diaphragmatic hernias masquerading as pleural effusion. *J. Pediatr.* 97:119–122, 1980.

22. Horbar, J. D. Neonatal GBS with right diaphragmatic hernia. *Hosp. Pract.* 15(Oct):142–147, 1980.

23. Harris, M. C. et al. Group B streptococcal septicemia and delayed-onset diaphragmatic hernia: a new clinical association. *Am. J. Dis. Child.* 135:723–725, 1981.

24. Edwards, M. S. et al. An etiologic shift in infantile osteomyelitis: the emergence of the group B streptococcus. *J. Pediatr.* 93:578–583, 1978

25. Baker, C. J. Group B streptococcal infections in neonates. *Pediatrics in Review* 1:5–15, 1979.

26. Hadeed, A. J. et al. Significance of transient post-natal hypothyroxinemia in premature infants with and without respiratory distress syndrome. *Pediatrics* 68:494–498, 1981.

27. Schönberger, W. et al. Transient hypothyroidism associated with prematurity, sepsis and respiratory distress. *Eur. J. Pediatr.* 132:85–92, 1979.

28. Neonatal bacteremia: diagnosis and management (editorial). *Br. Med. J.* 2:1385–1386, 1979.

29. Yeung, C. Y. Hypoglycemia in neonatal sepsis. *J. Pediatr.* 77:812–817, 1970.

30. Yeung, C. Y.; Lee, V. W. Y.; and Yeung, C. M. Glucose disappearance rate in neonatal infection. *J. Pediatr.* 82:486–489, 1973.

31. Leake, R. D.; Fisher, R. H., Jr.; and Oh, W. Rapid glucose disappearance in infants with infection. *Clin. Pediatr.* 20:397–401, 1981.

32. Shands, J. W., Jr.; Miller, V.; and Martin, H. The hypoglycemic activity of endotoxin. I: Occurrence in animals hyper-reactive to endotoxin. *Proc. Soc. Exp. Biol. Med.* 130:413–417, 1969.

33. James, T., and Blessa, M. Recurrent hyperglycemia associated with sepsis in a neonate. *Am. J. Dis. Child.* 133:645–646, 1979.

34. Feigin, R. D. et al. Inappropriate secretion of antidiuretic hormone (ADH) in children with bacterial meningitis. *Am. J. Clin. Nutr.* 30:1482–1484, 1977.

35. Rivers, R. P. A.; Forshing, M. L.; and Olver, R. P. Inappropriate secretion of antidiuretic hormone in infants with respiratory infections. *Arch. Dis. Child.* 56:358–363, 1981.

36. Gotoff, S. P., and Behrman, R. E. Neonatal septicemia. *J. Pediatr.* 76:142–153, 1970.

37. Corrigan, J. J. Thrombocytopenia: a laboratory sign of septicemia in infants and children. *J. Pediatr.* 85:219–221, 1974.

38. Zipursky, A., and Jaber, H. M. The haematology of bacterial infection in newborn infants. *Clin. Haematol.* 7:175–193, 1978.

39. Bell, M. J.; Ternberg, J. L.; and Bower, R. J. The microbial flora and antimicrobial therapy of neonatal peritonitis. *J. Pediatr. Surg.* 15:569–573, 1980.

40. Brill, P. W. et al. Osteomyelitis in a neonatal intensive care unit. *Radiology* 131:83–87, 1979.

41. Moss, T. J., and Pysher, T. J. Hepatic abscess in neonates. *Am. J. Dis. Child.* 135:726–728, 1981.

42. Daum, R. S., and Smith, A. L. Bacterial sepsis in the newborn. *Clin. Obstet. Gynecol.* 22:385–408, 1979.

43. Bowen, A. D. Hydrops of the gall-bladder and cholelithiasis in neonates (letter). *Acta Paediatr. Scand.* 71:839–841, 1982.

SEVEN

Traditional Sepsis Work-Up

It is comparatively recently that the majority of the risk and clinical factors described in chapters 4 and 5 have been used to initiate an investigation for sepsis. Approximately 30 years ago emphasis was directed toward the nonspecific nature of the signs indicating neonatal sepsis and meningitis.[1] A series of publications in the ensuing 10 to 15 years led to the frequent consideration of sepsis in the differential diagnosis for several different clinical circumstances.[2] In 1970, Gotoff and Behrman emphasized that "one must be willing to overdiagnose or misdiagnose" and that a presumptive diagnosis is made from three to five times as often as it is confirmed by blood cultures.[2] This statement undoubtedly led to what might be termed *overzealous investigation*. Their estimate was shown to be well short of the mark for subsequent years. For instance, it was shown in 1977 that as many as 23 babies were being investigated and treated with antibiotics for every baby who proved to have sepsis.[3] In the author's experience, the ratio of sepsis work-ups to proved cases of sepsis was approximately 11 to 1 (580 to 53) in an intensive care nursery.[4] This sepsis work-up usually consisted of culturing blood, CSF, and urine before initiating antibiotic therapy, but it is important to realize that "in the field" (rather than in academic centers), the cultures frequently were dispensed with and antibiotics started rather empirically.

Blood Cultures

In order to perform a satisfactory blood culture, it is necessary to minimize the possibility of contamination by organisms on the skin surface by cleaning the skin with an antiseptic agent. The best agents for this purpose are iodine or iodinated compounds, which should be allowed to act for at least 1 minute before proceeding.[5] If sterile gloves are not worn it may also be necessary to wipe the finger used to palpate a vein prior to inserting the needle.

Any large vein may be used to obtain blood. The amount of blood required to obtain a positive culture is not completely certain, but depends on the size of the inoculum.[6] As little as 0.5 ml or less can be used, although 1.0 ml generally is recommended.[5,6] Dietzman and colleagues found that a 0.2-ml specimen of blood is sufficient to detect 84% of *Escherichia coli* bacteremias.[7]

Until fairly recently the veins of choice were the external jugular or the femoral; however, the most suitable position for visualizing the external jugular vein requires rotation and extension of the neck, which may result in partial airway occlusion. In the well baby this position may not present a problem, but in the sick or preterm infant (who is more prone to sepsis) this could produce undesirable effects resulting from hypoxemia.[8] When performed correctly, sampling from the femoral vein is safer, but complications of poor technique include introduction of infection into the peritoneum (i.e., peritonitis) via the inguinal canal or into the hip joint (i.e., septic arthritis, osteomyelitis, or both).[9]

For these reasons, the antecubital vein or other large veins on the back of the hand or dorsum of the foot are used most frequently. An even more reliable source of blood is an umbilical artery catheter, particularly when it is inserted within the first 12 hours after delivery. The reliability of blood cultures taken from umbilical artery catheters inserted early in the neonatal period (i.e., first 9 hr) was documented by Cowett and co-workers.[10] It seems wise to wait approximately 30 minutes after insertion of a catheter before sampling blood for culture, so that any tendency to sample a transient bacteremia is lessened—although more rapid sampling did not produce false-positive results in the study by Cowett.[10] The usefulness of umbilical artery catheters is in contrast to that of umbilical vein catheters, in which a high percentage of false-positive blood cultures may be obtained.[5,11]

Although sampling blood from veins is the preferred method in most centers, capillary blood from heelsticks can provide a useful alternative.[12,13] This method of sampling has been found useful in at least two centers, but is more likely to provide false-negative results because of the decreased amount of blood used for culture. At least 50 colony forming units/ml blood would be required[6] and others have shown 54% of positive blood cultures contained 49 or less colony forming units.[7] There also may be false-positives, presumably due to contamination.

Another technique, which has generally been abandoned, is the use of umbilical cord blood cultures. Although this method is generally considered to yield an excessive number of positive cultures, a recent study disputes this opinion.[14] The authors of this recent report believe that meticulous and fastidious collection of umbilical cord blood cultures can provide a satisfactory alternative in those infants considered "at risk" at the time of delivery. They examined 200 cultures of 2-ml blood samples, 6 of which were positive. Three had delayed growth, two were considered contaminants and the remaining culture correlated with the infant's peripheral venous blood culture.[14]

Some controversy exists over how many blood cultures should be taken for reliable results. In general, it is not prudent to withhold antibiotic therapy if a neonate appears sick; therefore, a single blood culture is relied on. Although it may be desirable to obtain two blood cultures,[2] under most circumstances a single culture seems to be satisfactory.[15] In a retrospective study of 366 neonates, blood cultures were positive in 56, with 28 in neonates considered septicemic. In each of these septic infants, a single blood culture was satisfactory.[15] In the early stages of sepsis, a single culture using a small inoculum could produce an erroneous result.[6,7]

Another question that occurs occasionally is When may cultures safely be considered negative? The answer is reasonably well defined, although there is still some room for discussion. In a study by Pichichero and Todd it was shown that 96% of blood cultures are positive within 48 hours and 98% positive within 72 hours.[16] In the absence of clinical manifestations it seems reasonable to rely on the results at 48 hours. Some organisms may take longer to obtain a positive culture, but when this happens it raises the question of whether the organism is pathogenic or whether it is a contaminant. It seems safe to say that a blood culture is probably negative if there is no growth after 48 hours, almost certainly negative after 72 hours, and definitely negative if there is no growth at 1 week.

It may be worth remembering that some organisms formerly considered contaminants are almost certainly pathogenic for the very preterm infant, who is an immunocompromised host. Attempts should be made to grow both aerobic and anaerobic organisms. It has been suggested that the role of anaerobic bacteria in neonatal sepsis has been underestimated, but others have questioned this statement (see chapter 2). Enhanced growth of anaerobes may be achieved by using unvented blood culture bottles. Other methods for enhancing recovery of bacteria include antimicrobial inactivation (e.g., sodium polyanetholsulfonate, penicillinase) and hypertonic media.[5]

Cerebrospinal Fluid Culture

In most cases where evaluation is being performed on the basis of risk factors alone, it is probably reasonable to perform only blood cultures, because bacterial meningitis statistically is less likely within 48 hours of birth. In the presence of clinical signs, however, particularly after 48 hours, CSF should be obtained for culture in any infant suspected of having sepsis. Although it is sometimes stated that meningitis is directly related to the magnitude of bacteremia, in one study, 15% of babies had meningitis without bacteremia,[17] and a review suggests that a figure of 30% is not uncommon.[6] In general, the cell count on CSF will give a good indication of whether or not bacterial meningitis is present. Because this is not always the case,[17] it is important to send the CSF for culture in every case where sepsis is suspected. Sometimes only bacteria are seen in CSF early in the course of the illness. In the study of Visser and Hall, 21 samples of CSF could be analyzed from 39 neonates with meningitis, and only 12 of 21 had more than 25 cells/ mm^3.[17]

As with blood cultures, positive CSF cultures are usually indicated by growth within 72 hours. In most cases, both blood and CSF cultures will be positive, but sometimes only the CSF grows organisms.[17,18] In the presence of a positive CSF culture within 24 to 48 hours, the lumbar puncture may be worth repeating to document response to treatment, as persistently positive CSF cultures may indicate ventriculitis.[19,20]

Lumbar punctures, or spinal taps, may need to be performed with even more attention to detail than with blood cultures. Positioning of the baby can be critical, as excessive flexion of the trunk or neck may produce hypoxemia.[21] In some cases, the sitting position may be tolerated better.[22] The skin should be cleaned with an iodinated preparation; needles with stylets should be used.[22] Although it may be easier to use a scalp vein needle for this purpose,[23] needles without stylets carry the risk of introducing epithelial cells into the spinal canal with subsequent epidermoid tumors.[24] The needle should be short—1″ in length—to allow greater stability during manipulation.

When positive, culture of CSF provides a specific organism; however, examination of the CSF smear may show bacteria that can be identified with some certainty much more rapidly.[5] In a cooperative meningitis study, 80% of organisms were correctly identified on smear with Gram's stain prior to culture results.[19] This opportunity should not be wasted, although it is unlikely that the choice or duration of antibiotics will be influenced. The use of 5% sheep's blood agar plates is recommended for CSF cultures, because *Listeria* and group B streptococci (GBS) (two of the most common organisms producing meningitis) produce a characteristic hemolysis.[5]

Urine Culture

The value of urine cultures in the first days after delivery has been questioned, because it is very unusual to have positive cultures at this age.[25] The author's experience is similar in neonates during the first week after birth. There is little doubt, however, that urine is a valuable body fluid to examine later in the neonatal period, as there can be an association between urinary tract infection and sepsis in the neonate. This association seems to be more likely in boys[6,26]; in girls it may relate to urinary tract abnormalities.[26] As noted in chapter 5, jaundice seems to be a frequent accompanying sign with urinary tract infection. In a recent study, sepsis was documented in 31% of neonates with urinary tract infection and abnormalities of the urinary system were found in 45% of the girls.[26]

For many years urinary tract infection was probably overdiagnosed in the neonatal period, because the usual method of collection was a bag specimen and bag specimens are now considered notoriously unreliable.[5,27,28] It should be noted, however, that a negative culture of "bagged" urine can be reassuring.[29] The preferred method of obtaining urine for culture is by suprapubic bladder aspiration, or bladder tap.[30] The reliability of this technique recently has been enhanced by transillumination[31] and real-time ultrasound. Ultrasound examination of the head is the primary focus for such equipment in the neonate, but many other parts of the body can be examined and a full or partially filled bladder can be readily documented.

The alternative technique for obtaining urine is "mid-stream" or "clean catch," which *can* be done in neonates, particularly in boys, but requires patience and quick reflexes!

Superficial Cultures

Information obtained from cultures of skin surfaces, umbilicus, or gastric aspirate do not indicate sepsis or meningitis, but may provide information that a baby has been exposed to certain organisms.[2,5,6] It may even be reasonable to say that a baby has been contaminated by these organisms, although *colonized* seems a better term. Some authors persist in using superficial cultures (i.e., same organism from 3 sites) as an indication of neonatal sepsis, but it is doubtful that this is adequate evidence to make a diagnosis of sepsis. In a study from South Africa, a large number of superficial cultures were positive in preterm infants, but only 3% of the babies had documented sepsis.[32]

If superficial cultures are obtained, the limitations of interpretation should be remembered; however, it may be possible to use the information under certain conditions. Pharyngeal cultures may allow the identification of neonates at risk for infection, as colonization with certain kinds of organism may protect against other, more virulent bacteria, whereas recovery of known pathogens places an infant at particular risk.[33] If antibiotics are given before transfer, but laboratory tests indicate infection, superficial cultures (e.g., GBS) may aid in management decisions. Similarly in the presence of pneumonia, tracheal aspirate cultures seem very valuable and other superficial cultures might help to support this diagnosis[34]; however, they do not indicate either sepsis or meningitis.

References

1. Parmalee, A. H. *Management of the newborn*. Chicago: Year Book Medical Publishers, 1952, pp. 336–341.

2. Gotoff, S. P., and Behrman, R. E. Neonatal septicemia. *J. Pediatr.* 76:142–153, 1970.

3. Hammerschlag, M. R. et al. Patterns of use of antibiotics in two newborn nurseries. *N. Engl. J. Med.* 295:1268–1269, 1977.

4. Philip, A. G. S. Detection of neonatal sepsis of late onset. *J.A.M.A.* 247:489–492, 1982.

5. Marks, M. I., and Welch, D. F. Diagnosis of bacterial infections of the newborn infant. *Clin. Perinatol.* 8:537–558, 1981.

6. Daum, R. S., and Smith, A. L. Bacterial sepsis in the newborn. *Clin. Obstet. Gynecol.* 22:385–408, 1979.

7. Dietzman, D. E.; Fischer, G. W.; and Schoenknecht, F. D. Neonatal *Escherichia coli* septicemia—bacterial counts in blood. *J. Pediatr.* 85:128–130, 1974.

8. Long, J. G.; Philip, A. G. S.; and Lucey, J. F. Excessive handling as a cause of hypoxemia. *Pediatrics* 65:203–207, 1980.

9. Asnes, R. S., and Arendar, G. S. Septic arthritis of the hip: a complication of femoral venipuncture. *Pediatrics* 38:387–389, 1966.

10. Cowett, R. M. et al. Reliability of bacterial culture of blood obtained from an umbilical artery catheter. *J. Pediatr.* 88:1035–1036, 1976.

11. Anagnostakis, D. et al. Risk of infection associated with umbilical vein catheterization: a prospective study in 75 newborn infants. *J. Pediatr.* 86:759–765, 1975.

12. Mangurten, H. H., and Lebeau, L. J. Diagnosis of neonatal bacteremia by a microblood culture technique. *J. Pediatr.* 90:990–992, 1977.

13. Knudson, R. P., and Alden, E. R. Neonatal heelstick blood culture. *Pediatrics* 65:505–507, 1980.

14. Polin, J. I. et al. Use of umbilical cord blood culture for detection of neonatal bacteremia. *Obstet. Gynecol.* 57:233–237, 1981.

15. Franciosi, R. A., and Favara, B. E. A single blood culture for confirmation of the diagnosis of neonatal septicemia. *Am. J. Clin. Pathol.* 57:215–219, 1972.

16. Pichichero, M. E., and Todd, J. K. Detection of neonatal bacteremia. *J. Pediatr.* 94:958–965, 1979.

17. Visser, V. E., and Hall, R. T. Lumbar puncture in the evaluation of suspected neonatal sepsis. *J. Pediatr.* 96:1063–1067, 1980.

18. Overall, J. C. Neonatal bacterial meningitis: analysis of predisposing factors and outcome compared with matched control subjects. *J. Pediatr.* 76:499–511, 1970.

19. McCracken, G. H., Jr., and Mize, S. G. A controlled study of intrathecal antibiotic therapy in gram negative enteric meningitis of infancy: report of the Neonatal Meningitis Co-operative Study Group. *J. Pediatr.* 89:66–72, 1976.

20. Hill, A.; Shackelford, G. D.; and Volpe, J. J. Ventriculitis with neonatal bacterial meningitis: identification by real-time ultrasound. *J. Pediatr.* 99:133–136, 1981.

21. Weisman, L. E.; Merenstein, G. B.; and Steenbarger, J. R. The effect of lumbar puncture position in sick neonates. *Am. J. Dis. Child.* 137:1077–1079, 1983.

22. Stevens, D. C.; Jose, J. H.; and Schreiner, R. L. Lumbar puncture in the neonate. *Resident Staff Physician* 26 (Sept):34–36, 1980.

23. Greensher, J. et al. Lumbar puncture in the neonate: a simplified technique. *J. Pediatr.* 78:1034–1035, 1971.

24. Shaywitz, B. A. Epidermoid spinal cord tumors and previous lumbar punctures. *J. Pediatr.* 80:638–640, 1972.

25. Visser, V. E., and Hall, R. T. Urine culture in the evaluation of suspected neonatal sepsis. *J. Pediatr.* 94:635–638, 1979.

26. Ginsburg, C. M., and McCracken, G. H., Jr. Urinary tract infections in young infants. *Pediatrics* 69:409–412, 1982.

27. Braude, H. et al. Cell and bacterial counts in the urine of normal infants and children. *Br. Med. J.* 4:697–701, 1967.

28. Newman, C. G.; O'Neill, P.; and Parker, A. Pyuria in infancy and the role of suprapubic aspiration of urine in diagnosis of infection of the urinary tract. *Br. Med. J.* 2:277–279, 1967.

29. Moncrieff, M. et al. Asymptomatic bacteriuria in healthy preterm babies. *Arch. Dis. Child.* 55:723–725, 1980.

30. Nelson, J. D., and Peters, P. C. Suprapubic aspiration of urine in premature and term infants. *Pediatrics* 36:132–134, 1965.

31. Kuhns, L. R. Bladder transillumination to facilitate bladder puncture (letter). *J. Pediatr.* 91:850, 1977.

32. Higgs, S. C.; Malan, A. F.; and Heese, H. de V. The perinatal infective environment and infants of very low birth weight. *S. Afr. Med. J.* 51:621–623, 1977.

33. Sprunt, K.; Leidy, G.; and Redman, W. Abnormal colonization of neonates in an intensive care unit: means of identifying neonates at risk of infection. *Pediatr. Res.* 12:998–1002, 1978.

34. Sherman, M. P. et al. Tracheal aspiration and its clinical correlates in the diagnosis of congenital pneumonia. *Pediatrics* 65:258–263, 1980.

E I G H T

Rapid, Useful, Nonspecific Diagnostic Tests

Leukocyte Counts

Earlier this century, a number of authors attested to the value of the leukocyte count in diagnosing neonatal sepsis.[1,2] Until very recently, however, the prevailing opinion was that the white blood cell and differential counts were of little value in the diagnosis of neonatal sepsis. This opinion was largely because many babies with apparently normal leukocyte counts had documented sepsis. On the other hand, many babies with leukopenia or neutropenia or both—and some with leukophilia, neutrophilia, or both—proved to have sepsis. A major 1974 review of neonatal sepsis stated that the leukocyte count is "usually unrevealing or uninterpretable"[3]; as recently as 1979, it was considered that "peripheral white blood cell counts are generally not reliable in the diagnosis of newborn sepsis."[4]

While it may be true that one cannot rely on leukocyte counts, abnormal counts can be quite informative and helpful. In particular, the immature/total neutrophil (I/T) ratio has proved to be a sensitive though nonspecific indicator of neonatal sepsis. In the author's experience, the combination of leukopenia (WBC counts $< 5000/mm^3$) and an increased I/T ratio (≥ 0.2) is highly predictive of neonatal sepsis.[5,6]

Current interest in the diagnostic importance of the leukocyte count (or counts) stems from the work of Xanthou[7,8] as well as that of Haider[9] and Gregory and Hey.[10] Zipursky and colleagues have suggested that the morphology of the cells as well as the total number of immature cells is more important than the absolute neutrophil count.[11-13] Manroe and co-workers emphasized the importance of both the presence of immature, or band, forms and the sensitivity of the I/T ratio in detecting neonatal sepsis.[14,15] The levels above which this I/T ratio are to be considered abnormal will alter its specificity, but values ⩾ 0.2 to 0.3 are highly predictive of sepsis (see Appendix table 7).[16,17] Very high values (⩾ 0.8) have been correlated with a depleted neutrophil storage pool in the bone marrow by Christensen and colleagues.[17]

The earlier work suggested that absolute neutrophil counts were helpful.[7-10] Although there is little doubt that an absolute neutropenia (particularly < 1000/mm³) is strongly suggestive of infection,[14,17,18] in the author's experience, neither absolute neutrophil counts nor absolute band counts are particularly sensitive tests for detecting neonatal sepsis (see Appendix table 7).

Other neutrophil ratios have been used—in particular, the band/ poly, or immature/mature neutrophil, ratio as described by Kuchler and colleagues,[19] Zipursky and Jaber,[13] and Christensen and co-workers.[17] There really is no difference between the origin of an immature/mature ratio and that of the I/T ratio, but the latter has the advantage of falling between 0 and 1. Another apparent advantage of the I/T ratio is that it does not appear to be significantly influenced by birth weight or gestational age, in contrast to other types of leukocyte count (see Appendix table 8). Some noninfected, very low birth weight infants can have very low total leukocyte counts (see Appendix Figure 1) for reasons that are not clear.

Another approach to the use of leukocyte counts in diagnosing neonatal sepsis is to perform repeat counts in the first 12 to 24 hours after birth. Several authors have observed that there is usually an increase in both total leukocyte and absolute neutrophil counts in the first 8 to 12 hours after birth.[7,11,15] Consequently, a decrease in these counts at such an age may be taken as evidence of sepsis.[20]

The morphologic neutrophil abnormalities described as suggestive of sepsis are Döhle's bodies, toxic granulation, and vacuolation,[12,13] but more recent experience has cast doubt on the specificity of these findings.[21] Taken with other suggestive findings, morphologic abnormalities of the neutrophils may point toward infection, but should not be relied on in isolation.

A number of potentially confusing factors in interpreting WBC counts should be mentioned. Manroe and colleagues found that neutrophil counts can be outside the normal range for 24 hours or more in response to maternal hypertension, maternal fever, neonatal asphyxia, and periventricular hemorrhage.[15] This effect of asphyxia was confirmed by Merlob and co-workers.[22] Two groups have shown increased counts when heelstick (capillary) measurements were compared with determinations on venous or arterial samples.[23,24]

Even without allowing for these confounding variables, some leukocyte counts are very sensitive (see Appendix table 7) and others quite predictive. Special attention should be drawn to leukopenia ($<$ 5000/mm) in combination with an elevated I/T ratio ($\geq$ 0.2). In a study by the author of 524 infants investigated in the first week after birth, 22 had this combination.[6] Of the 22, 15 had documented sepsis (total with sepsis was 41) and 4 infants had documented bacterial pneumonia, indicating that this combination is highly predictive for bacterial infection (see Appendix table 15).

Perhaps the most important point is that the leukocyte count has the major advantage of being readily available in any hospital. Thus, it provides the basis for diagnosing neonatal sepsis, remembering both that a normal count does not exclude infection and that it requires proper interpretation.[15,24]

Acute-Phase Reactants

Just as there has been a good deal of skepticism about the value of leukocyte counts in diagnosing sepsis, there seems to be even less enthusiasm in the United States for employing other laboratory tests. Most of these other tests are considered unhelpful or unreliable in making a diagnosis of neonatal sepsis. For example, two recent chapters on neonatal sepsis in textbooks devoted to infectious diseases in children make no mention of the possible value of acute-phase proteins,[25,26] although one text does mention the erythrocyte sedimentation rate (ESR).[26]

Despite this apparent gap in our knowledge, there is an increasing amount of information about the value of acute-phase reactants in di-

Table 8.1.
*Normal Values and Probable Range of Several Acute-Phase Reactants
During Systemic Infection in Neonates*

Reactant	Normal level		Usual range with systemic infection
	1–2 Days	3–7 Days	
ESR (mm/1hr)	< 3	< 10	10–40
Fibrinogen (mg/dl)	<250	<400	300–600
C-Reactive protein (mg/dl)	< 1.6	< 1.0	3.0–20.0
Haptoglobin (mg/dl)	< 25	< 50	25–200
α1-Acid glycoprotein (mg/dl)	< 50	< 75	50–250

agnosing neonatal sepsis, most of which comes from Scandinavia and Europe. Acute phase proteins seem to be useful in diagnosis; they may be even more helpful in following the course of the disease. The following discussion will be limited to those acute-phase reactants (or acute-phase proteins) that have been documented as useful in the diagnosis of infection in the neonate, although others may also be altered (usually increased) and subsequently prove useful.

The following acute-phase reactants will be considered:

1. Erythrocyte sedimentation rate (principally reflecting fibrinogen)
2. Fibrinogen
3. C-Reactive protein
4. Haptoglobin
5. α_1-Acid glycoprotein (orosomucoid)

Although all these proteins may show discernible changes, C-reactive protein shows the most dramatic increase in concentration: it can be approximately 100 times the usual concentration, as opposed to the two- to threefold increase with most other clinically useful acute-phase proteins.[27] The normal values and likely range during infection are provided in table 8.1.

In addition, some components of complement (e.g., C3 and C9) are increased with infection, as is α_1-antitrypsin; transferrin and prealbumin seem to be negative acute-phase reactants (i.e., they decrease with infection).[27a]

Erythrocyte Sedimentation Rate

Although sedimentation of erythrocytes had been noted for many years, the first clinical application of erythrocyte sedimentation rate (ESR) was by Fåhreus, who was looking for a test to document pregnancy.[28] At about the same time, Westergren used it in tuberculosis.[29] Subsequently, Landau described the application of a microtechnique for pediatric use.[30] In 1970, Evans and colleagues described the application of this micro-ESR to the evaluation of infection in neonates.[31] An even simpler method was described in 1975 by Adler and Denton using a microhematocrit capillary tube, which is filled to the brim, sealed at one end, and placed in a vertical position for 1 hour.[32] The volume of blood required is approximately 75 µl, as opposed to 2 to 3 ml for the Westergren method. They termed this a *mini-ESR,* although the values probably differ little from the micro-ESR method.[32] Thus, perhaps the simplest solution is to refer to the *mESR.*

A number of factors influence ESR; however, the major factor producing an accelerated rate—given a hematocrit in the normal range—is an increase in plasma fibrinogen.[33] This is probably because fibrinogen is a rather spindle-shaped molecule[34] and because the surface charge on the erythrocytes may be altered to favor rouleaux formation.[35] Personal observations indicate that in the neonate, increased fibrinogen is the primary determinant of an increased mESR.

Several studies now indicate that the mESR can be a useful adjunct in the diagnosis of neonatal infection.[5,6,32,36,37] It is important to realize that a normal mESR may be common in the early stages of infection (or in face of disseminated intravascular coagulation); however, the presence of an increased mESR is suggestive of infection. Although in the author's experience, the level of 15 mm/hr proved most useful for diagnosing infection, a lower level may be considered abnormal in the first 2 or 3 days after delivery.[5,6] Some details are provided in the Appendix (table 9; figure 3).

Normal levels have been documented as 0 to 3 mm/hr in the first 2 or 3 days, with a gradual rise during the first 2 to 4 weeks to a 95th percentile of 15 to 17 mm/hr.[32] At the other extreme, maximal values are determined by the hematocrit level. In a 75-mm capillary tube the sedimentation will be limited by the hematocrit (e.g., hematocrit of 60% = maximum mESR of 30 mm/hr, 50% = 37 mm/hr, and so on).

Fibrinogen

The principal role of fibrinogen is in blood coagulation, but it has been shown to be an acute-phase reactant in a number of adult inflammatory responses.[38] Relier and colleagues in Paris have demonstrated the acute-phase response of this protein in neonatal infection in several papers.[39–41] They suggest fibrinogen levels above 250 mg/dl during the first 2 to 3 days and above 400 mg/dl on subsequent days are suggestive of neonatal infection. More recent evidence suggests that fibrinogen levels may be increased in other sick neonates who are not infected[42]; in another report, only 5 of 16 proved cases of infection had elevated fibrinogen levels on the day of clinical onset.[13]

The value of fibrinogen levels in neonatal sepsis needs further verification, but one report from Paris suggests that infection sensitive to the antibiotics chosen will have a return to normal fibrinogen levels within 3 days, whereas persistently elevated levels may indicate antibiotic resistance.[41] The mean levels are demonstrated in table 8.2. In another report from France, 69% (40) of 58 infected neonates had elevated fibrinogen levels, in contrast to 83% (48) who had high orosomucoid (α_1-acid glycoprotein). Orosomucoid was increased and fibrinogen normal in 13 infants; the reverse was true in 5 infants.[43]

C-Reactive Protein

The acute-phase protein that has attracted the most attention in recent years is C-reactive protein (CRP). As mentioned earlier, the enormous increase in CRP levels with infection (or other inflammatory disorders) over levels found normally (as much as 100-fold, or even 1000-fold in adults) makes this a particularly fascinating protein to study.[27,35,44–46]

C-Reactive protein was discovered in 1930 by Tillett and Francis during studies on pneumococcal disease.[47] The name *C-reactive protein* was derived from the fact that during acute illness, there was a

Table 8.2.

Mean Levels (mg/dl) of Fibrinogen in Control and Infected Infants

Age (in days)	Control (n = 30)	Infected, sensitive organism (n = 17)	Infected, resistant organism (n = 12)
1	235	453	440
2	274	447	469
3	306	379	464
4	323	298	438
5	328	307	412
6	318	313	392
7	277	280	269

Modified from E. de Gamarra et al. Surveillance du taux de fibrinogène chez le nouveau-né:intérêt au cours de l'évolution des infections bactériennes par contamination d'origine maternelle. *Arch. Fr. Pediatr.* 37:163–166, 1980.

precipitation reaction of patients' sera with the C-polysaccharide fraction of the pneumococcus. Subsequently, in pediatrics, the detection of CRP was found to be helpful in diagnosing rheumatic fever; however, with the decline in incidence of rheumatic fever, most physicians abandoned this test.

For many years, CRP was considered to be normally not present in the serum of healthy individuals. As methods of assay became more sensitive, CRP was found to be present in low concentration in most people. Like most other proteins, the site of production is the liver, which was shown convincingly by Kushner and Feldman.[48] More recently, it has been suggested that CRP production is triggered by way of leukocytes or macrophages. The release of interleukin-1 (also called endogenous pyrogen and other terms) may be the stimulus to production of CRP; prostaglandins also may mediate the synthesis of CRP and other acute-phase proteins.[27] C-Reactive protein probably is the most rapidly responsive acute-phase protein, with significant increases occurring within 6 to 8 hours of the insult producing experimental inflammation.[48]

Although CRP levels increase in response to a wide variety of inflammatory or necrotic stimuli, the most likely reason for an increase in the neonate is infection.[49] This response was initially described by

Felix and colleagues in 1966, using a semiquantitative method.[50] Subsequently, radial immunodiffusion was used to document increases in levels of CRP in infants with infection, first by Saxstad and colleagues[51] and later by Sabel and Hanson.[52]

One of the problems with older studies of CRP levels using the radial immunodiffusion method was the time needed to obtain a result—approximately 24 hours—which limited its usefulness as a practical diagnostic aid. With the advent of a rapid, semiquantitative latex agglutination test, results can be obtained within 10 minutes. In a more recent study by Sabel and Wadsworth, 89% (16 of 18) of neonates with bacterial sepsis had an initial increase in the level of CRP.[53] The author's experience with this test (see Appendix table 13) suggests that a somewhat lower percentage will have increased levels when first evaluated, but that the percentage will later rise. There is also evidence to suggest that different bacteria will initiate different responses, with *Escherichia coli* perhaps being consistently the most likely to cause an increase in CRP levels.[52,53] Profound neutropenia or leukopenia as seen with group B streptococcal infection may attenuate the response, and failure to respond in the face of documented sepsis can be a poor prognostic sign.[54]

Other studies support the usefulness of CRP levels in the diagnosis of neonatal sepsis. In one study from Spain, 100% of neonates with systemic infection had initially increased levels of CRP.[55] In another study from South Africa, 8 of 10 neonates with sepsis, meningitis, or both had a positive latex agglutination test for CRP when first evaluated.[56] Further evidence is provided by a German study, which showed a positive latex agglutination CRP test in 14 of 15 neonates with documented sepsis, in 14 of 22 with probable infection, and in 6 of 73 uninfected neonates.[57]

Caution in overinterpreting an elevated CRP level has recently been proposed by Ainbender and colleagues because, in some other disorders (e.g., meconium aspiration syndrome) there may be a modest increase in CRP levels, presumably because of an inflammatory response.[58] Because the latex agglutination test does not provide a specific level of CRP, it may be best to screen with a rapid, inexpensive and simple test like the latex agglutination test and proceed to a quantitative test if it is positive. A number of nephelometric techniques can now provide rapid—within 1 hour—determinations.[59,60]

In addition to the diagnostic use of CRP, CRP levels can be very useful in determining response to treatment and can be incorporated into management decisions on when to stop antibiotics.[27a] In particular, it should be noted that in cases of meningitis, the only three cases to relapse in the series of Sabel and Hanson had elevated CRP levels when antibiotics were stopped.[52] The value of using CRP to decide duration of antibiotics was recently given more support by the study of Squire and colleagues.[61] A major advantage in studying CRP sequentially is that because it is found in low concentration in adults as well as neonates, blood transfusion should not cause any difficulty in interpretation. Evidence supporting the value of CRP in diagnosing and following the course of neonatal sepsis continues to appear.[62-64]

Haptoglobin

Discovered by Polonovski and Jayle in 1938, haptoglobin (Hp) was named for its ability to bind free hemoglobin released into plasma from red cell breakdown.[65] Consequently, Hp has been used primarily as a measure of hemolysis in older persons, as the hemoglobin-haptoglobin complex is removed by the reticuloendothelial system with depletion of plasma Hp levels. In addition to this function, Hp also was found to be an acute-phase reactant[66] and has been used with other acute-phase reactants in the assessment of several disorders in adults, particularly rheumatoid arthritis.[67]

For many years, Hp was considered to be present rarely in neonates, at least in the first few days after birth.[68] In the late sixties and early seventies, however, it became apparent that Hp could be demonstrated in almost every baby, but usually in greatly decreased concentrations[69-71] This discovery led to the suggestion that even normal (i.e., adult) levels might indicate infection,[70] which was demonstrated more than a decade ago by Salmi in his large review.[72]

From other experimental (i.e., animal) evidence, Hp appears to be slower to respond than CRP.[27,35,45,46,73] This response seems to be true in the human newborn, where elevation of Hp levels appears to be more akin to increased mESR. Thus, by itself Hp is not a very sensitive diagnostic tool early in the course of sepsis, but when levels are increased, Hp is apparently quite predictive (see Appendix tables 11 and 13).

There are several different methods of estimating Hp levels.[68–72,74] Older methods relied on its ability to bind hemoglobin and were measured as hemoglobin binding capacity (methemoglobin apparently being the most sensitive). Radial immunodiffusion has the limitation of time needed to obtain the result (as mentioned for CRP), although there are now nephelometric techniques that can provide rapid results. In addition, a latex agglutination test is available, which takes slightly longer than the latex agglutination test for CRP because a short—15 minutes—incubation period is required. Interestingly, in my own experience, some infants with sepsis had positive Hp latex agglutination tests but negative CRP latex agglutination tests at initial evaluation; no specific organism was associated with this finding.[5]

Until the present time, few studies have incorporated Hp levels into the assessment of neonatal sepsis: in addition to the studies quoted,[5,72] one Japanese study[75] and one German[57] attest that Hp usually increases in neonates with infection. Because Hp levels tend to increase postnatally (in contrast to CRP) and might also be influenced by blood transfusion, minor increases need to be interpreted with caution.

α_1-Acid Glycoprotein

Among the other acute-phase reactants, the only one that has attracted attention for use in the diagnosis of neonatal infection is α_1-acid glycoprotein (α_1-AGP), which is frequently referred to as orosomucoid in Europe and Scandinavia. This protein was discovered more recently than the others and, although its function is still being elucidated, its structure was established in 1973.[76] In that same year, the first description of its use in neonates was reported from Japan.[77] Subsequent reports from Japan,[75] France,[78] and Germany[57] of studies in neonatal infection were varying in their enthusiasm. In 1981 Sann and colleagues provided extensive experience with the use of α_1-AGP in neonates with and without infection, using the technique of laser nephelometry.[43] (As noted earlier, this method is much more rapid than radial immunodiffusion.) They suggested that there is a rapid increase in levels during the first week after birth, independent of gestational age, with a more gradual rise to adult levels by 10 months of age. They also suggested that first-day levels were lower in preterm neonates. The author has confirmed that gestational age influences the level of α_1-AGP in cord blood and first-day samples (see Appendix fig. 4).[79]

Sann and colleagues demonstrated that in infants with severe bacterial infections, initially elevated levels of α_1-AGP were seen in 85%.[43] In those with increased levels, the evolution of serum concentrations followed the clinical course. Slight elevation of α_1-AGP levels was seen in approximately 25% of 630 sick neonates without demonstrable infection.[43] Failure of an infected infant to increase levels of α_1-AGP may have prognostic significance.[54] In contrast to the usual increase seen in survivors, neonates with infection who died frequently failed to respond.[43]

The rapidity of the response of α_1-AGP to infection may lie somewhere between CRP and Hp, although this response possibly may be variable depending on the infecting organism. Increasing levels of α_1-AGP could be of some help in distinguishing respiratory distress syndrome (RDS) from pneumonia. In a preliminary report, low levels of α_1-AGP were noted in the cord blood of neonates who subsequently developed RDS.[80] This might be attributed to the effect of gestational age on levels of α_1-AGP (alluded to earlier), because more recent evidence suggests that approximately 14% of patients with RDS have initially high α_1-AGP levels.[43] In contrast, neonates with "congenital" pneumonia may have initially increased levels[49]; levels are likely to rise significantly over the next few days in cases of pneumonia, but would probably decline in RDS.[43] Further studies are needed to confirm or refute this suggestion.

Combinations of Tests

It is apparent from the preceding discussion that the majority of studies that describe the value of diagnostic tests for neonatal sepsis focus on a single test. Obviously, if a single test was always positive with sepsis and there were few false-positives, it would be reasonable to rely on a single test; this is not possible with the tests currently available.

In attempting to evaluate a test or combination of tests, it is useful to consider the information that can be derived from table 8.3. It is also

Table 8.3.
Method for Evaluating Diagnostic Tests for Neonatal Sepsis

	Disease (sepsis) present	**Disease absent**
Test positive	a	b
Test negative	c	d

Sensitivity = how frequently the test is positive if the disease is present; expressed by

$$\frac{a}{a + c}$$

Specificity = how frequently the test is negative if the disease is absent; expressed by

$$\frac{d}{b + d}$$

Positive predictive value (or accuracy) = how frequently the disease is present when the test is positive; expressed by

$$\frac{a}{a + b}$$

Negative predictive value (or accuracy = how frequently the disease is absent when the test is negative: expressed by

$$\frac{d}{c + d}$$

Efficiency = how frequently the test predicts correctly (i.e., false-positives and false-negatives excluded); expressed by

$$\frac{a + d}{a + b + c + d}$$

important to know how much reliance could be placed on the various tests at the time that the diagnosis of sepsis was suspected and cultures were sent. In this way, the value of each test can be assessed under the clinical circumstances usually encountered.[81–83]

In order to judge which attributes are most valuable in a given disorder, Galen and Gambino[83] have outlined several principles. They believe that the highest *sensitivity* is desired if (1) the disease is serious and should not be missed, (2) the disease is treatable, and (3) false-positives do not produce serious psychological or economic trauma. The highest *specificity* is needed if the disease is serious but not treatable. They believe further that a high *positive predictive value* is essential if treatment of false-positives might have serious consequences; highest *efficiency* is desired if (1) the disease is serious but treatable, and (2) false-positives and false-negatives are equally serious or damaging.

Applying these principles, neonatal sepsis must be considered a serious, but treatable, disease whose diagnosis should not be missed.

Although "overtreatment" of false-positives may not have serious consequences for the individual baby, it could be a problem over time. Under such circumstances, it is desirable to have a sensitive test with as high a positive predictive value as possible.[83] Because incidence or prevalence may influence positive predictive value, this indicator should be compared with the incidence or prevalence in the group under investigation.

In general, tests used to diagnose neonatal sepsis have not been subjected to the kind of analysis illustrated by table 8.3. This is particularly true for combinations of tests, although some authors have looked at several tests in investigating sepsis, without using them in combination. The author's evaluation of several tests singly and in combination is provided in the Appendix (table 13). When two or more of five tests were positive, both sensitivity and positive predictive value were greatest. These tests were leukocyte count $< 5000/mm^3$, I/T ratio ≥ 0.2, CRP latex agglutination test positive, Hp latex agglutination test positive, and mESR ≥ 15 mm/hr.

Few other reports have considered tests in combination. One of these was published by Gotoh and colleagues in Japan and described an acute-phase reactants score, which used the combination of Hp, CRP, and α_1-AGP levels.[75] This was considered a screening test, but at the time, the measurement technique for these proteins was radial immunodiffusion, which requires 18 to 24 hours to complete. Such a delay would not allow results to be incorporated into clinical decisions about antibiotics (at least not at the time of initial investigation); however, techniques now available could allow this acute-phase reactants score to be reevaluated, with the possibility of clinical application.

The only other scoring system of which I am aware was reported from Mexico, and combined CRP, α_1-antitrypsin, and α_1-AGP levels, mESR, and platelet count. After evaluating 56 neonates, Vargas and colleagues concluded that platelet count and mESR were sufficient to diagnose sepsis.[84] While this may be true of the population seen in Mexico City, the limited evidence in that study and conflicting evidence from other studies suggests that further evaluation is required before applying their finding to North American, European, Scandinavian, or other populations.

Although combining tests has been used very infrequently, *comparison* of tests has attracted some attention. With regard to the leukocyte count and acute-phase reactants, several recent studies have provided comparisons. Two of these were mentioned earlier[56,57]; one compared quantitative measurements of CRP, Hp, and α_1-AGP levels.[57] Although CRP, in particular, and Hp were considered useful, α_1-AGP did not appear to discriminate between healthy and infected neonates. In the second study, mESR, CRP latex agglutination, and total leukocyte count were compared.[56] The CRP latex agglutination test had the greatest predictive value and sensitivity. The mESR was significantly raised in all cases of documented neonatal infection, but tended to remain elevated despite clinical response to therapy.

Squire and colleagues[61] also evaluated a number of tests, including leukocyte counts, mESR, and CRP levels and concluded that no test was completely satisfactory, but agreed with others[52,53] that CRP levels may help to follow the course of the illness. The study of Spector and co-workers suggests that a combination of clinical features and leukocyte counts is the best method of diagnosing infection and deciding when to use antibiotics.[85] They reached this conclusion, however, by applying the most useful features retrospectively. Prospective evaluation needs to be carried out and might prove useful.

In another recent study, Töllner developed a scoring system for diagnosing neonatal sepsis by combining the blood count with clinical features.[86] The score was derived from retrospective analysis of 83 neonates with septicemia and was then applied prospectively in 39 neonates with septicemia as well as in other babies. This method may have merit, although intra-, or peri-, ventricular hemorrhage may produce high scores.[86]

Endotoxemia

The detection of endotoxin was successfully applied to the examination of urine and cerebrospinal fluid in the seventies. The test used was the limulus amebocyte lysate (LAL) test, which uses as the reagent an extract prepared by lysis of the amebocyte blood cell of the horseshoe crab, *Limulus polyphemus*. By incubating the test sample with an equal volume of reagent in a test tube, presence of endotoxin is indicated when gelation of the mixture is noted while gently inverting the tube. Other techniques for detecting endotoxin have been described more recently.[87]

A positive latex LAL test suggests the presence of endotoxin and by inference indicates a gram-negative infection. This test was used in neonates to detect meningitis caused by gram-negative organisms.[88,89] For many years, detection of endotoxin in plasma was considered unreliable because of the presence of substances that inhibited the gelation reaction. Because the only way to remove these inhibitor substances seemed to be a chloroform extraction procedure that required large samples of blood (5–15 ml), the possibility of detecting neonatal endotoxemia seemed remote. It was recently shown, however, first in adults[90] and then in neonates,[87] that the inhibitor substances can be largely inactivated by heating. This simplified the approach to detection of endotoxin in plasma.

In two communications in 1981, Scheifele and colleagues in Vancouver suggested that the clinical picture of neonatal sepsis might be initiated by the presence of endotoxin alone, without the demonstration of bacteremia.[87,91] The implication of their findings was that many neonates may be exposed to infection (or the effects of gram-negative infection) without having demonstrable evidence on blood culture. In fact, during the first 7 days after delivery, one third of septic-appearing but nonbacteremic infants apparently had endotoxemia.

In infants older than 1 week, there was a stronger association between gram-negative bacteremia and endotoxemia; but of considerable interest (and possibly greater significance) was the presence of several cases (6 of 10) of necrotizing enterocolitis among those with a false-positive LAL test. In this regard it is interesting to speculate on the significance of false-positive CRP latex agglutination tests noted in the evaluation of infants suspected of having sepsis. Endotoxin is known to stimulate an acute-phase response, including an increase in the levels of CRP.[92] Thus, if endotoxemia is considered a manifestation of sepsis, many of the false-positive CRP tests may no longer be false.

References

1. Washburn, A. H. Blood cells in healthy young infants: a study of 608 differential leukocyte counts, with final report on 908 total leukocyte counts. *Am. J. Dis. Child.* 50:413–430, 1935.

2. McLaren-Todd, R. Septicemia of the newborn: a clinical study of fifteen cases. *Arch. Dis. Child.* 23:102–106, 1948.

3. Wilson, H. D., and Eichenwald, H. F. Sepsis neonatorum. *Pediatr. Clin. North Am.* 21:571–582, 1974.

4. Daum, R. S., and Smith, A. L. Bacterial sepsis in the newborn. *Clin. Obstet. Gynecol.* 22:385–408, 1979.

5. Philip, A. G. S., and Hewitt, J. R. Early diagnosis of neonatal sepsis. *Pediatrics* 65:1036–1041, 1980.

6. Philip, A. G. S. Detection of neonatal sepsis of late onset. *J.A.M.A.* 247:489–492, 1982.

7. Xanthou, M. Leucocyte blood picture in healthy full-term and premature babies during neonatal period. *Arch. Dis. Child.* 45:242–249, 1970.

8. Xanthou, M. Leucocyte blood picture in ill newborn babies. *Arch. Dis. Child.* 47:741–747, 1972.

9. Haider, S. A. Polymorphonuclear leucocyte count in diagnosis of infection in the newborn. *Arch. Dis. Child.* 47:394–395, 1972.

10. Gregory, J., and Hey, E. Blood neutrophil response to bacterial infection in the first month of life. *Arch. Dis. Child.* 47:747–753, 1972.

11. Akenzua, G. I. et al. Neutrophil and band counts in the diagnosis of neonatal infections. *Pediatrics* 54:38–42, 1974.

12. Zipursky, A. et al. The hematology of bacterial infections in premature infants. *Pediatrics* 57:839–853, 1976.

13. Zipursky, A., and Jaber, H. M. The haematology of bacterial infection in newborn infants. *Clin. Haematol.* 7:175–193, 1978.

14. Manroe, B. L. et al. The differential leukocyte count in the assessment and outcome of early-onset neonatal group B streptococcal disease. *J. Pediatr.* 91:632–637, 1977.

15. Manroe, B. L. et al. The neonatal blood cell count in health and disease. I. Reference values for neutrophilic cells. *J. Pediatr.* 95:89–98, 1979.

16. Boyle, R. J. et al. Early identification of sepsis in infants with respiratory distress. *Pediatrics* 62:744–750, 1978.

17. Christensen, R. D.; Bradley, P. P.; and Rothstein, G. The leukocyte left shift in clinical and experimental neonatal sepsis. *J. Pediatr.* 98:101–105, 1981.

18. Squire, E.; Favara, B.; and Todd, J. Diagnosis of neonatal bacterial infection: hematologic and pathologic findings in fatal and nonfatal cases. *Pediatrics* 64:60–64, 1979.

19. Kuchler, H.; Fricker, H.; and Gugler, E. La formule sanguine dans le diagnostic précoce de la septicémie du nouveau-né. *Helv. Paediatr. Acta* 31:33–46, 1976.

20. Töllner, U., and Pohlandt, F. Septicemia in the newborn due to gram-negative bacilli: risk factors, clinical symptoms and hematologic changes. *Eur. J. Pediatr.* 123:243–254, 1976.

21. Leslie, G. I.; Scurr, R. D.; and Barr, P. A. Early-onset bacterial pneumonia: a comparison with severe hyaline membrane disease. *Aust. Paediatr. J.* 17:202–206, 1981.

22. Merlob, P. et al. The differential leukocyte in full-term newborn infants with meconium aspiration and neonatal asphyxia. *Acta Paediatr. Scand.* 69:779–780, 1980.

23. Christensen, R. D., and Rothstein, G. Pitfalls in the interpretation of leukocyte counts of newborn infants. *Am. J. Clin. Pathol.* 72:608–611, 1979.

24. Peevy, K. J.; Grant, P. H.; and Hoff, C. J. Capillary venous differences in neonatal neutrophil values. *Am. J. Dis. Child.* 136:357–358, 1982.

25. Krugman, S., and Katz, S. L. Sepsis in the newborn. In *Infectious diseases of children,* 7th edition. St. Louis: C. V. Mosby Co., 1981, pp. 208–219.

26. McCracken, G. H., Jr. *Perinatal bacterial diseases.* In *Textbook of pediatric infectious disease.* Philadelphia: W. B. Saunders, 1981, pp. 747–768.

27. Gewurz, H. Biology of C-reactive protein and the acute phase response. *Hosp. Pract.* 17(June):67–81, 1982.

27a. Philip, A. G. S. Acute phase proteins in neonatal infection (editorial). *J. Pediatr.,* in press.

28. Fåhreus, R. The suspension stability of the blood. *Acta Med. Scand.* 55:1–228, 1921.

29. Westergren, A. Studies of the suspension stability of the blood in pulmonary tuberculosis. *Acta Med. Scand.* 54:247–282, 1921.

30. Landau, A. Microsedimentation (Linzenmeier-Raunert method). *Am. J. Dis. Child.* 45:691–734, 1933.

31. Evans, H. E.; Glass, L.; and Mercado, C. The micro-erythrocyte sedimentation rate in newborn infants. *J. Pediatr.* 76:448–451, 1970.

32. Adler, S. M., and Denton, R. L. The erythrocyte sedimentation rate in the newborn period. *J. Pediatr.* 86:942–948, 1975.

33. Talstad, I., and Hangen, H. F. The relationship between the erythrocyte sedimentation rate (ESR) and plasma proteins in clinical materials and models. *Scand. J. Lab. Invest.* 39:519–524, 1979.

34. Doolittle, R. F. Fibrinogen and fibrin. *Sci. Am.* 245:126–135, 1981.

35. Kushner, I. The acute phase reactants and the erythrocyte sedimentation rate. In *Textbook of rheumatology,* eds. W. N. Kelley et al. Philadelphia: W. B. Saunders Co., 1981, pp. 669–676.

36. Ibsen, K. K. et al. The value of the micromethod erythrocyte sedimentation rate in the diagnosis of infections in newborns. *Scand. J. Infect. Dis.* 23(Suppl.):143–145, 1980.

37. Moodley, G. P. The microerythrocyte sedimentation rate in black neonates and children. Part I: Its value in suspected neonatal infection. *S. Afr. Med. J.* 59:943–945, 1981.

38. Kindmark, C. O. Sequential changes in plasma proteins in various acute diseases. In *Plasma protein turnover;* eds. R. Bianchi; G. Mariani; and A. S. McFarlane. Baltimore: University Park Press, 1976, pp. 395–402.

39. Relier, J. P. et al. Intérêt de la mesure du taux de fibrinogène dans les infections néonatales par contamination maternelle. *Arch. Fr. Pediatr.* 33:109–120, 1976.

40. Relier, J. P., and de Bethmann, O. Diagnosis of neonatal sepsis via materno-fetal transmission. *Antibiot. Chemother.* 21:146–150, 1976.

41. de Gamarra, E. et al. Surveillance du taux de fibrinogène chez le nouveau-né: intérêt au cours de l'évolution des infections bactériennes par contamination d'origine maternelle. *Arch. Fr. Pediatr.* 37:163–166, 1980.

42. Coulombel, L. et al. Intérêt des données hématologiques pour le diagnostic d'infection materno-foetale. Etude prospective chez le nouveau-né. *Arch. Fr. Pediatr.* 37:385–391, 1980.

43. Sann, L. et al. Serum orosomucoid concentration in newborn infants. *Eur. J. Pediatr.* 136:181–185, 1981.

44. Pepys, M. B. C-reactive protein fifty years on. *Lancet* 1:653–657, 1981.

45. Kushner, I.; Gewurz, H.; and Benson, M. D. C-reactive protein and the acute phase response. *J. Lab. Clin. Med.* 97:739–749, 1981.

46. Gewurz, H. et al. C-reactive protein and the acute-phase response. *Adv. Intern. Med.* 27:345–372, 1982.

47. Tillett, W. S., and Francis, T. Serological reactions in pneumonia with a non-protein somatic fraction of pneumococcus. *J. Exp. Med.* 52:561–571, 1930.

48. Kushner, I., and Feldman, G. Control of the acute phase response: demonstration of C-reactive protein synthesis and secretion by hepatocytes during acute inflammation in the rabbit. *J. Exp. Med.* 148:466–477, 1978.

49. Hanson, L. A. et al. The diagnostic value of C-reactive protein. *Pediatr. Infect. Dis.* 2:87–90, 1983.

50. Felix, N. S.; Nakajima, H.; and Kagan, B. M. Serum C-reactive protein in infections during the first six months of life. *Pediatrics* 37:270–277, 1966.

51. Saxstad, J.; Nilsson, L. A.; and Hanson, L. A. C-reactive protein in serum from infants as determined with immunodiffusion techniques. II: Infants with various infections. *Acta Paediatr. Scand.* 59:676–680, 1970.

52. Sabel, K. G., and Hanson, L. A. The clinical usefulness of C-reactive protein (CRP). Determination in bacterial meningitis and septicemia in infancy. *Acta Paediatr. Scand.* 63:381–388, 1974.

53. Sabel, K. G., and Wadsworth, C. C-reactive protein (CRP) in early diagnosis of neonatal septicemia. *Acta Paediatr. Scand.* 68:825–831, 1979.

54. Philip, A. G. S. The protective effect of acute phase reactants in neonatal sepsis. *Acta Paediatr. Scand.* 68:481–483, 1979.

55. Matesanz, J. L. et al. Valor diagnóstico de la proteína C reactiva en la sepsis neonatal. *An. Esp. Pediatr.* 13:671–678, 1980.

56. Moodley, G. P. The micro-erythrocyte sedimentation rate in black neonates and children. Part II: A comparative study of the micro-erythrocyte sedimentation rate, C-reactive protein test and total white cell count. *S. Afr. Med. J.* 60:545–547, 1981.

57. Pilars de Pilar, E. et al. Akute phase-proteine bei früh-und neugeborenen. *Klin. Pädiatr.* 192:45–50, 1980.

58. Ainbender, E. et al. Serum C-reactive protein and problems of the newborn. *J. Pediatr.* 101:438–440, 1982.

59. Harmoinen, A.; Hallström, O.; and Grönroos, P. Rapid quantitative determination of C-reactive protein using laser nephelometer. *Scand. J. Clin. Lab. Invest.* 40:293–295, 1980.

60. Gill, C. W. et al. An evaluation of a C-reactive protein assay using a rate immuno-nephelometric procedure. *Am. J. Clin. Pathol.* 75:50–55, 1981.

61. Squire, E. N. et al. Criteria for the discontinuation of antibiotic therapy during presumptive treatment of suspected neonatal infection. *Pediatr. Infect. Dis.* 1:85–90, 1982.

62. Alt, R. et al. Intérêt de la C-réactive protéine dans les infections bactériennes néonatales. *Arch. Fr. Pediatr.* 39:811–813, 1982.

63. Speer, C.; Bruns, A.; and Gahr, M. Sequential determination of CRP, α_1-antitrypsin and haptoglobin in neonatal septicaemia. *Acta Paediatr. Scand.* 72:679–683, 1983.

64. Sann, L. et al. α_1-Acid glycoprotein and C-reactive protein in the evolution of bacterial infection of neonates (abstr.). *Pediatr. Res.* 18:285A, 1984.

65. Polonovski, M., and Jayle, M. F. Existence dans le plasma sanguin d'une substance activant l'action peroxydasique de l'hémoglobine. *Compte. Rendu. Soc. Biol.* 129:457–460, 1938.

66. Kauder, E., and Mauer, A. M. The physiology and clinical significance of haptoglobin. *J. Pediatr.* 59:286–295, 1961.

67. McConkey, B. et al. Effects of gold, dapsone and prednisone on serum C-reactive protein and haptoglobin and the erythrocyte sedimentation rate in rheumatoid arthritis. *Ann. Rheum. Dis.* 38:141–144, 1979.

68. Nyman, M. Serum haptoglobin: methodological and clinical studies. *Scand. J. Clin. Lab. Invest.* 11(Suppl. 39):1–169, 1959.

69. Drakowa, D. The relation of serum haptoglobin levels to age and sex in healthy children. *Arch. Immunol. Ther. Exp.* 14:47–55, 1966.

70. Philip, A. G. S. Haptoglobins in the newborn. I. Full term infants. *Biol. Neonate* 19:185–193, 1971.

71. Philip, A. G. S. Haptoglobins in the newborn. II. Low birth weight babies. *Biol. Neonate* 19:332–338, 1971.

72. Salmi, T. T. Haptoglobin levels in the plasma of newborn infants: with special reference to infections. *Acta Paediatr. Scand.* (Suppl. 241):1–55, 1973.

73. Aronsen, K. F. et al. Sequential changes of plasma proteins after surgical trauma. *Scand. J. Clin. Lab. Invest.* 29(Suppl. 124):127–131, 1972.

74. Tarukoski, P. H. Quantitative spectrophotometric determination of haptoglobin. *Scand. J. Clin. Lab. Invest.* 18:80–86, 1966.

75. Gotoh, H. et al. Evaluation of APR-score (acute phase reactants score) as a screening test of neonatal infection. *Jpn. Neonatal Soc. J.* 10:78–84, 1974.

76. Schmid, K. et al. Structure of α_1-acid glycoprotein: the complete amino acid sequence, multiple amino acid substitutions, and homology with the immunoglobulins. *Biochemistry* 12:2711–2724, 1973.

77. Gotoh, H. et al. Diagnostic significance of serum orosomucoid level in bacterial infections during neonatal period. *Acta Paediatr. Scand.* 62:629–632, 1973.

78. Sann, L. et al. Etude de l'orosomucoide chez le nouveau-né: interêt dans le diagnostic des infections bactériennes. *Arch. Fr. Pediatr.* 33:961–971, 1976.

79. Philip, A. G. S., and Hewitt, J. R. α_1-Acid glycoprotein in the neonate with and without infection. *Biol. Neonate* 43:118–124, 1983.

80. Lee, S. K.; Thibeault, D. W.; and Heiner, D. C. α_1-Antitrypsin and α_1-acid glycoprotein levels in the cord blood and amniotic fluid of infants with respiratory distress syndrome. *Pediatr. Res.* 12:775–777, 1978.

81. Card, W. I., and Emerson, P. A. Test reduction: I. Introduction and review of published work. *Br. Med. J.* 281:543–545, 1980.

82. Feinstein, A. R. Clinical biostatistics XXXI: on the sensitivity, specificity and discrimination of diagnostic tests. *Clin. Pharmacol. Ther.* 17:104–116, 1975.

83. Galen, R. S., and Gambino, S. R. *Beyond normality: the predictive value and efficiency of medical diagnosis.* New York: John Wiley and Sons, 1975, p. 129.

84. Vargas, O. A. et al. Evaluación de algunas pruebas de laboratorio para el diagnóstico de septicemia en el neonato. *Bol. Méd. Hosp. Infant. Méx.* 37:1135–1140, 1980.

85. Spector, S. A.; Ticknor, W.; and Grossman, M. Study of the usefulness of clinical and hematologic findings in the diagnosis of neonatal bacterial infections. *Clin. Pediatr.* 20:385–392, 1981.

86. Töllner, U. Early diagnosis of septicemia in the newborn: clinical studies and sepsis score. *Eur. J. Pediatr.* 138:331–337, 1982.

87. Scheifele, D. W.; Melton, P.; and Whitchelo, V. Evaluation of the *Limulus* test for endotoxemia in neonates with suspected sepsis. *J. Pediatr.* 98:899–903, 1981.

88. McCracken, G. H., and Sarff, L. D. Endotoxin in cerebrospinal fluid:

detection in neonates with bacterial meningitis. *J.A.M.A.* 235:617–620, 1976.

89. Dyson, D., and Cassady, G. Use of *Limulus* lysate for detecting gram-negative neonatal meningitis. *Pediatrics* 58:105–109, 1976.

90. DuBose, D. A. et al. Comparison of plasma extraction techniques in preparation of samples for endotoxin testing by the *Limulus* amoebocyte lysate test. *J. Clin. Microbiol.* 11:68–72, 1980.

91. Scheifele, D. W.; Melton, P. W.; and Ebelt, V. Endotoxinaemia per se as cause of neonatal morbidity (letter). *Lancet* 1:337, 1981.

92. Yen-Watson, B., and Kushner, I. Rabbit CRP response to endotoxin administration: dose response relationship and kinetics. *Proc. Soc. Exp. Biol. Med.* 146:1132–1136, 1974.

N I N E

Diagnostic Tests of Doubtful Value

Platelet Count

One of the problems of test interpretation is that the retrospective analysis of a disease may suggest tests that do not prove valuable when they are evaluated prospectively. Another problem is whether from one hospital to another, like is being compared with like. These points are emphasized with respect to platelet counts because when infants with sepsis are evaluated, many of them will have thrombocytopenia at some point in their illness. For instance, Zipursky and Jaber indicate that thrombocytopenia was seen in 13 of 24 neonates with sepsis, but in only 3 was it seen on the day of onset.[1] Thus, the finding of thrombocytopenia may be important in supporting a diagnosis of neonatal sepsis, but it appears to be a late finding or confirmatory of severe infection. In one recent study, 10 of 16 neonates with positive blood or CSF cultures or both had thrombocytopenia ($< 100,000/mm^3$), but the mean time from initial symptoms to thrombocytopenia was 21.5 hours.[2]

Thrombocytopenia originally was considered a useful marker of neonatal infection, and in some centers it appears to be a common finding with neonatal sepsis.[3-5] The author's experience, however, is in accord with other recent studies, which indicate that thrombocytopenia is a late feature.[1,2,6,7] In other words, the presence of thrombocytopenia does not seem to be a useful test for early diagnosis of sepsis.

The mechanism of production of thrombocytopenia generally has been thought to relate to bone marrow—in this case megakaryocyte—

suppression, or to increased peripheral consumption or destruction (e.g., aggregation, lysis, or disseminated intravascular coagulation.[1] One recent investigation suggests that there may be an immune basis for the thrombocytopenia associated with neonatal sepsis.[8] Platelet-associated immunoglobulin was increased over normal levels in 8 of 9 infants with bacterial sepsis and in 6 of 8 infants with severe viral infection. The return to normal platelet counts takes an average of 7 days, with a range of from 1 to 10 days; it may closely follow clinical improvements.[2,8]

Of course, thrombocytopenia can occur for other reasons. For instance, infants born to mothers with pregnancy-induced hypertension had thrombocytopenia ($< 150,000/mm^3$) significantly more frequently than did controls.[9]

Gastric Aspirate Smear and Culture

One diagnostic method that has been used extensively is the smear— and culture—of fluid obtained by gastric aspiration shortly after birth. The presence of large numbers of white blood cells or many bacteria of a single type on smear seems to be of aid, because it provides some information fairly quickly—in contrast to culture. The information is somewhat limited, however, indicating only that the baby has been *exposed* to infection, not that the baby is infected. The usual reason for obtaining the gastric aspirate is that the baby is suspected to have come from an infected environment, on the basis of prolonged rupture of membranes, foul-smelling amniotic fluid, unexplained preterm labor, or other predisposing risk factors. Therefore, a positive gastric aspirate smear (usually more than 5 WBC/high-power field or presence of bacteria) provides confirmation of the suspect environment, a fact pointed out by Gotoff and Behrman many years ago.[10]

The initial studies using this technique suggested that it was a useful indicator of neonatal infection[11,12]; however, it was subsequently shown that the source of the leukocytes was maternal, not fetal.[13] In recent years, a number of reports have questioned the value of this test,[14–16] and the author's personal experience suggests that this test has limited usefulness.[17] If one considers only neonates with early-onset sepsis, not noninfected infants, it may appear valuable. For instance,

Boyle and colleagues showed that 5 of 7 infants with sepsis had positive gastric aspirate smears; 23 smears were positive in 83 noninfected babies.[15] On the other hand, Mims and co-workers examined 197 consecutive gastric aspirate smears from newborns: 27 smears were considered positive, but none of the infants was septic.[14]

Umbilical Cord Histology

Abnormal umbilical cord histology, like positive gastric aspirate smears, has been considered a reflection of amniotic fluid infection. The purpose of umbilical cord examination is to find a perivascular inflammatory response, which presumably is indicative of funisitis. If such a response is found, the implication is that the infant is at particularly high risk for infection. The actual yield of neonatal sepsis under these circumstances, however, is comparatively low: the so-called inflammatory response may be initiated by asphyxia.[18]

Because preparation of the sections and histologic interpretation require the help of a pathologist, there are limitations of time, availability, practicality, and interpretation. After initial enthusiasm, both Blanc[19] and Benirschke[20] seem to have abandoned this method of evaluation. The method's utility was again proposed in 1970[21,22]; more recently it also has been reported to give valuable information concerning infection.[23] The reader may judge the usefulness of umbilical cord histology by examining table 9.1.

Immunoglobulin M Levels

There have been several reports of the course of immunoglobulin M levels during acute bacterial infection in the neonate. Although an increase in IgM levels after 48 to 72 hours is frequently observed, an increase within 24 hours of the onset of illness is very uncommon. Because of this, IgM levels do not seem to be helpful in making an early diagnosis of sepsis. In addition, because IgM apparently is more of a "subacute" phase reactant than an acute-phase reactant, following IgM levels through the course of an illness is unlikely to help determine the efficacy of treatment.

Table 9.1.

Correlation of Abnormal Umbilical Cord Histology with Evidence of Infection

Group	Total examined	Total with funisitis
Proved infection*	10	4
Probable infection	11	6
Doubtful infection	52	12
No infection	111	5

Modified from J. Kérisit et al. L'examen histologique extemporané du cordon ombilical: un procédé fiable pour l'appreciation du risque inféctieux néonatal. *J. Gynecol. Obstet. Biol. Reprod.* (Paris) 10:45–49, 1981.

*Positive blood, CSF cultures, or both.

The initial enthusiasm for the determination of IgM levels occurred around 1969[24–26]; even then Korones and colleagues noted the delayed response. In 1973, Salmi reiterated that while haptoglobin responded acutely, IgM was slow to respond.[27] Personal observations confirm that an early increase in IgM levels is unusual, although gram-negative infections usually are accompanied by a subsequent rise. Immunoglobulin M levels may take as long as 3 or 4 weeks to drop.[28,29]

Nitroblue Tetrazolium Reduction Test

The neutrophils of patients with bacterial infections were noted to reduce the dye nitroblue tetrazolium (NBT) more rapidly than did the neutrophils of normal controls. The value of this test has been disputed in both adults and neonates.[1,30] It was suggested that neutrophils of low birth weight infants gave higher values and caused difficulties of interpretation.[31,32] Because of these problems, the test was not considered useful; however, it was proposed that most of the problems were related to heparin administration and that if careful standardization of the amount of heparin was employed, many problems could be eliminated.[32]

A further modification of the NBT test recently appeared in the French literature, where it was suggested as a good screening test for neonatal infection.[33] The NBT test was performed on 44 controls aged 1 to 6 days, as well as on 72 infants less than 48 hours of age being investigated for infection. One hundred cells were scored from 0 to 3, for a maximum score of 300. Infants with proved or suspected infection usually had scores greater than 100, in contrast to the low scores obtained in controls and noninfected neonates.[33] It is important to understand that the test cannot be performed in the presence of neutropenia. It also has limitations in differentiating babies with sepsis and respiratory distress from those with respiratory distress syndrome (i.e., hyaline membrane disease).[15,34] For instance, in the study of Boyle and colleagues, of the seven septic infants in whom the NBT test was performed, four were so neutropenic that the test could not be performed and only one of the other three was outside the range seen in respiratory distress syndrome.[15]

Buffy Coat Smear

The evaluation of the buffy coat smear to document neonatal bacteremia was first described in 1976.[35] The principle of the test is that bacteria engulfed by neutrophils can be demonstrated on a stained smear of the buffy coat. As with the NBT test, the test is difficult to perform in the presence of leukopenia, neutropenia, or both. The whole slide needs to be examined before declaring the test negative, which can take up to half an hour of careful study. On the other hand, the finding of engulfed bacteria can be quite rapid, so that, from a practical point of view, a positive test may be helpful. A negative test needs to be interpreted with caution; many times the test cannot be interpreted because of neutropenia.

Several authors have mentioned using the buffy coat smear in the evaluation of neonatal sepsis,[15] but there has been no large-scale documentation of the value of this test in the neonatal period. Faden found positive buffy coat smears in 7 of 10 infants with documented sepsis.[35] Four of the seven died. Boyle and colleagues were able to document four positive smears in four infants with sepsis and found no positives in 105 noninfected babies.[15] Larger numbers of infected babies are needed for study. A note of caution was sounded in an adult study, when positive tests were seen sporadically in acutely ill patients with fever but without demonstrable bacteremia; repeatedly positive findings in the buffy coat correlated with persistent bacteremia.[36] At this point, there is not enough information available on which to base a valid judgment in the neonate. It is possible that the use of acridine orange stain may improve the ability to detect bacteria in buffy coat smears.[37]

One advantage that a positive buffy coat smear seems to give is a preliminary identification of the causative organism. More recently, another technique has been described that also requires confirmation: the use of a direct blood smear for bacteria, which may provide equally reliable information.[38] Extra- and intracellular bacteria could be demonstrated in peripheral blood smears in 17 of 19 septic infants; there were 9 false-positives.[38]

Other Smears

Placental Smear

One technique that seems to be a cross between cord histology and a direct blood smear is the use of a placental smear. This technique has been used widely in France and involves using a slide to obtain a smear for bacteriologic examination, after stripping off the membranes.[39]

Ear Canal Fluid Smear

Some time ago, when the value of examining the gastric aspirate was considered greater than it is today, it was proposed that fluid in the external auditory canal might provide a useful source for detecting infection.[40] The rationale behind this proposal was that in infants transferred to an intensive care nursery, who might have had the gastric fluid discarded, the fluid in the ear canal could provide evidence of the organism to which the baby had been exposed. Examination of the ear canal fluid does not seem to be widely done or particularly helpful.

References

1. Zipursky, A., and Jaber, H. M. The haematology of bacterial infection in newborn infants. *Clin. Haematol.* 7:175–193, 1978.

2. Modanlou, H. D., and Ortiz, O. B. Thrombocytopenia in neonatal infection. *Clin. Pediatr.* 20:402–407, 1981.

3. Corrigan, J. J. Thrombocytopenia: a laboratory sign of septicemia in infants and children. *J. Pediatr.* 85:219–221, 1974.

4. Tchernia, G. et al. Thrombopénies et infections bacteriénnes néonatales. *Nouv. Rev. Fr. Hematol.* 15:484–495, 1975.

5. Jasso, G. L., and Vargas, O. A. Thrombocitopenia como indice de septicemia en el recien nacido. *Gac. Méd. Méx.* 111:317–320, 1976.

6. Spector, S. A.; Ticknor, W.; and Grossman, M. Study of the usefulness of clinical and hematologic findings in the diagnosis of neonatal bacterial infections. *Clin. Pediatr.* 20:385–392, 1981.

7. Töllner, U. Early diagnosis of septicemia in the newborn: clinical studies and sepsis score. *Eur. J. Pediatr.* 138:331–337, 1982.

8. Tate, D. Y. et al. Immune thrombocytopenia in severe neonatal infections. *J. Pediatr.* 98:449–453, 1981.

9. Brazy, J. E.; Grimm, J. K.; and Little, V. A. Neonatal manifestations of severe maternal hypertension occurring before the thirty-sixth week of pregnancy. *J. Pediatr.* 100:265–271, 1982.

10. Gotoff, S. P., and Behrman, R. E. Neonatal septicemia. *J. Pediatr.* 76:142–153, 1970.

11. Ramos, A., and Stern, L. Relationship of premature rupture of the membranes to gastric fluid aspirate in the newborn. *Am. J. Obstet. Gynecol.* 105:1247–1251, 1969.

12. Yeung, C. Y., and Tam, A. S. Y. Gastric aspirate findings in neonatal pneumonia. *Arch. Dis. Child.* 47:735–740, 1972.

13. Vasan, U. et al. Origin of gastric aspirate polymorphonuclear leukocytes in infants born after prolonged rupture of membranes. *J. Pediatr.* 91:69–72, 1977.

14. Mims, L. C. et al. Predicting neonatal infections by evaluation of the gastric aspirate: a study in two hundred and seven patients. *Am. J. Obstet. Gynecol.* 114:232–238, 1972.

15. Boyle, R. J. et al. Early identification of sepsis in infants with respiratory distress. *Pediatrics* 62:744–750, 1978.

16. Roos, P. J. et al. The bacteriological environment of preterm infants. *S. Afr. Med. J.* 57:347–350, 1980.

17. Philip, A. G. S., and Hewitt, J. R. Early diagnosis of neonatal sepsis. *Pediatrics* 65:1036–1041, 1980.

18. Salem, F. A., and Thadepalli, H. Microbial invasion of the placenta, cord and membranes during active labor: a not infrequent finding, usually unassociated with clinical sepsis of the newborn. *Clin. Pediatr.* 18:50–52, 1979.

19. Blanc, W. A. Pathways of fetal and early neonatal infection: viral placentitis, bacterial and fungal chorioamnionitis. *J. Pediatr.* 59:473–495, 1961.

20. Benirschke, K. Routes and types of infection in the fetus and newborn. *Am. J. Dis. Child.* 99:714–721, 1960.

21. Overbach, A. M.; Daniel, S. J.; and Cassady, G. The value of umbilical cord histology in the management of potential perinatal infection. *J. Pediatr.* 76:22–31, 1970.

22. Olding, L. Value of placentitis as a sign of intra-uterine infection in human subjects: a morphological, bacteriological, clinical and statistical study. *Acta Pathol. Microbiol. Scand.* [A] 78:256–264, 1970.

23. Kérisit, J. et al. L'examen histologique extemporané du cordon ombilical: un procédé fiable pour l'appreciation du risque inféctieux néonatal. *J. Gynecol. Obstet. Biol. Reprod.* (Paris) 10:45–49, 1981.

24. Korones, S. B. et al. Neonatal IgM response to acute infection. *J. Pediatr.* 75(Part 2):1261–1270, 1969.

25. Blankenship, W. J. et al. Serum gamma-M globulin responses in acute neonatal infections and their diagnostic significance. *J. Pediatr.* 75:1271–1281, 1969.

26. Khan, W. N. et al. Immunoglobulin M determinations in neonates and infants as an adjunct to the diagnosis of infection. *J. Pediatr.* 75:1282–1286, 1969.

27. Salmi, T. T. Haptoglobin levels in the plasma of newborn infants: with special reference to infections. *Acta Paediatr. Scand.* Suppl. 241:1–55, 1973.

28. Haider, S. A. Serum IgM in diagnosis of infection in the newborn. *Arch. Dis. Child.* 47:382–393, 1972.

29. Bueno, M. et al. Bacterial infections in the newborn. *Helv. Paediatr. Acta* 32:479–486, 1977.

30. Steigbigel, R. T.; Johnson, P. K.; and Remington, J. S. The nitroblue tetrazolium reduction test versus conventional hematology in the diagnosis of bacterial infection. *N. Engl. J. Med.* 290:235–238, 1974.

31. Park, B. H. The use and limitations of the nitroblue tetrazolium test as a diagnostic aid. *J. Pediatr.* 78:376–378, 1971.

32. Chandler, B. D. et al. Nitroblue tetrazolium test in neonates. *J. Pediatr.* 92:638–640, 1978.

33. Dalens, B. et al. Dépistage rapide de l'infection néonatale par le test au nitroblue de tétrazolium réalisé selon des modalités nouvelles. *J. Gynecol. Obstet. Biol. Reprod.* 10:39–43, 1981.

34. Kalpaktsoglou, P. K. et al. Evaluation of nitroblue tetrazolium test in low birth-weight infants. *J. Pediatr.* 84:441–443, 1974.

35. Faden, H. S. Early diagnosis of neonatal bacteremia by buffy-coat examination. *J. Pediatr.* 88:1032–1034, 1976.

36. Studer, J-P.; Glauser, M. P.; and Schapira, M. Value of examining buffy coats for intragranulocytic micro-organisms in patients with fever. *Br. Med. J.* 1:85–86, 1979.

37. Kleiman, M. B. et al. Acridine orange stain of buffy coat smears in the newborn (abstr.) *Pediatr. Res.* 17:273A, 1983.

38. Storm, W. Early detection of bacteremia by peripheral blood smears in critically ill newborns. *Acta Paediatr. Scand.* 70:415–416, 1981.

39. Sarrut, S. Intérêt du frottis amniotique dans le dépistage de l'infection néonatale. *Méd. Inf.* 81:525–535, 1974.

40. Scanlon, J. The early detection of neonatal sepsis by examination of liquid obtained from the external ear canal. *J. Pediatr.* 79:247–249, 1971.

T E N

Rapid, Specific Diagnostic Tests

Countercurrent Immunoelectrophoresis

The diagnosis of sepsis is only made definitively by culturing bacterial organisms from blood; the tests described in the preceding chapters are nonspecific indicators of the disease state. The usefulness of such nonspecific indicators is that the information may be available rapidly and can be incorporated into decisions about antibiotic treatment. It is apparent that even more information would be available if a specific diagnosis could be made quickly and easily. The first indication that this might be possible occurred in the mid-seventies with the introduction of countercurrent immunoelectrophoresis (CIE).[1] Application of CIE to the diagnosis of neonatal sepsis occurred in the late seventies.[2-4]

The principle of CIE is the ability of bacterial antigen in various body fluids to react with an antiserum (i.e., antibody)—prepared against the specific antigen—to form a complex. The complex can be displayed by passing an electric current through the medium holding the fluid (or gel) so that a precipitation ring (or curve) can be quantitated. The demonstration of the antigen (using the precipitin lines) does not prove absolutely that infection is present, but is strongly supportive evidence, which may be available within 1 to 2 hours. Most information in the neonatal period is confined to demonstration of group B streptococcal (GBS) antigen.[2-4]

Other antigens available for use with CIE are *Haemophilus influenzae* type b,[5] certain strains of pneumococci, meningococci, and K_1 antigen of *Escherichia coli*. Apart from the *E. coli* antigen, the others will be encountered infrequently with neonatal infection. At present,

121

antisera for detection of *E. coli* are not commercially available but there is antigenic cross-reaction between *E. coli* K_1 antigen and meningococcus group B capsular polysaccharide.[6]

One of the advantages of tests used to detect antigen is that they may remain positive after the onset of administration of antimicrobials. In some cases, antigen can be demonstrated for many days. A disadvantage of the tests carried out several years ago was the lack of reliability of the antisera; although this remains a potential problem, the currently available antisera seem to give reliable results.

In the study of Stechenberg and colleagues, when body fluids of 61 infants with GBS infection were examined with CIE, at least one of the urine, CSF, or blood samples was positive in 95% of cases.[3] Concentrated urine seemed to be the most reliable body fluid with 81% of samples being positive. The results of Baker and co-workers were even more striking, with 100% of 67 patients with GBS bacteremia, meningitis, or both having one or more of the three body fluid samples positive at the time of admission; urine concentrated 50-fold gave 96% positive results—100% in cases of bacteremia.[7] They also confirmed that the addition of 4% dextran improved the sensitivity of the test and made the immunoprecipitin lines sharper and more easily read.

The mean duration of antigenuria (urine being the most reliable body fluid) in the study of Baker and colleagues was 5.2 days (range = 1–30 days) in cases of GBS bacteremia and 22.4 days (range = 1–75 days) in cases of GBS meningitis.[7] Despite the greater yield from urine, it may be advisable to send serum and CSF for evaluation in any case where GBS infection is suspected. Particularly in the infant who is poorly perfused, time can be a factor: there may be delay in obtaining a specimen of urine and further delay in concentrating the urine, as well as the time it takes to perform the test. In such circumstances, a positive test may be obtained more quickly with serum or CSF.

Latex Particle Agglutination Test

Antisera for use with CIE are prepared by injecting the antigen to be tested into an animal known to respond with antibody production. Whenever antisera are available for use with CIE, they should also be available to be incorporated into a latex particle agglutination (LPA) test. The major advantage of the LPA method of antigen detection is the rapidity with which it can be performed. Sample size can also be extremely small (approximately 20 μl). By adding a small drop of the antisera attached to polystyrene latex particles to the small sample, specific antigen can be detected by the resulting agglutination into clumps or granules. Not only can group-specific antisera be prepared, but type-specific antisera have also been produced.

Despite the simplicity of this technique, it seems to have given superior results when compared with CIE by several different observers.[8-11] For instance, Edwards and colleagues looked at the CSF of infants with type III GBS meningitis and showed 12 of 12 infants positive by LPA test and 11 of 12 positive by CIE on admission.[8] In subsequent evaluation of CSF while the infants received therapy, the LPA test was positive in 14 of 26 compared with 11 of 26 with CIE. Bromberger and co-workers also looked at infants with GBS infection not confined to meningitis.[9] The most striking finding was that in 11 newborns with GBS infection, unconcentrated urine gave 7 positive by LPA test but only 1 by CIE. With concentrated urine, all 11 were positive by LPA test, while 8 were positive using CIE.

In older infants, Ward and colleagues showed that the LPA test was somewhat superior to CIE in diagnosing *H. influenzae* type b infections.[5,12] The value of this antiserum in the neonatal period is somewhat limited, because even though there are a number of reports of infection in the neonatal period resulting from *H. influenzae*, they have been caused by type c or untypable strains (see chapter 2).

Another study of neonatal GBS infection was reported by Ingram and associates.[10] Once again, 100% of 18 infected neonates with urine available for concentration had a positive LPA test, and in most categories, the LPA test appeared more sensitive than CIE in detecting GBS antigen. More recent evaluation with a commercially available antiserum suggests that there may be considerable variability in the potency of antisera.[11] Some antisera give a high percentage of false-positive results, so that these possibilities should be kept in mind when interpreting results.

Enzyme-Linked Tests

The most generally available enzyme-linked test is referred to as ELISA, which stands for enzyme-linked immunosorbent assay. This test has been applied primarily to viral infections, but can also be applied to bacterial antigens.[13]

More recently, monoclonal antibodies produced by continuous cultures of hybrid myeloma cell lines have been used in an enzyme-linked inhibition assay to detect streptococcal antigen. In the study by Polin and Kennett, monoclonal antibodies specific for type II and type III GBS were available.[14] Type III GBS antigen was detected in CSF specimens from 11 culture-proved cases of GBS meningitis and in the knee aspirate from an infant with GBS septic arthritis. Five other CSF specimens from infants with meningitis caused by other bacterial organisms, as well as 10 other control samples were negative. Once again, the sample volume used was very small (approximately 25 µl), and the sensitivity of the test measured quantities of antigen 80 to 90 times less than that detected by CIE or LPA. A further refinement, providing a rapid answer, uses a technique called monoclonal antibody sandwich enzyme assay.[15] This assay has the advantage of having color production rather than color inhibition as the end point.

Another technique with potential application is the radioisotopic assay of enzymes. In particular, β-lactamase—which is produced by a number of pathogenic organisms—has been measured in blood, peritoneal, pleural, and cerebrospinal fluids.[16]

Other Tests

Coagglutination and Immunofluorescence

Coagglutination of *Staphylococcus aureus* may be almost as good as CIE in detecting several antigens associated with sepsis or meningitis in older children and there is a commercially available system for detecting GBS antigen (Phadebact), which may be helpful in neonates.[13] Immunofluorescence has been used mostly for viral infections,[13], but does not seem to have been frequently evaluated in bacterial infections occurring during the neonatal period, although GBS antigen has been detected.[17]

Gas-Liquid Chromatography

Although gas-liquid chromatography (GLC) is not always readily available, its use in detection of amniotic fluid infection has been noted earlier (see chapter 4) and the technique may be applicable to neonatal infection. The principle is that certain bacteria will produce volatile fatty acids that may provide patterns on GLC that are sufficiently specific to be diagnostic.

A presumptive anaerobic infection was described in a neonate in 1977,[18] and cases of meningitis caused by *Streptococcus pneumoniae* and *H. influenzae* have been detected using GLC on the spinal fluid, although the latter experience was primarily with dogs.[19]

Direct Examination

As noted under the section on buffy coat smears (chapter 9), direct examination of blood smears may provide considerable help, which can be fairly specific. The same holds true for examination of CSF.[13] As noted by others, the presence of gram-positive cocci in chains or gram-negative rods in the neonate can probably be called GBS or *E. coli,* respectively, with considerable confidence.[6] Similarly, small, gram-positive pleomorphic rods strongly suggest *Listeria* infection in this age group. Recently it has also been suggested that acridine-orange stain may improve diagnostic accuracy.[20]

References

1. Feigin, R. D. et al. Countercurrent immunoelectrophoresis of urine as well as of CSF and blood for diagnosis of bacterial meningitis. *J. Pediatr.* 89:773–775, 1976.

2. Edwards, M. S., and Baker, C. J. Prospective diagnosis of early onset group B streptococcal infection by countercurrent immunoelectrophoresis. *J. Pediatr.* 94:286–288, 1979.

3. Stechenberg, B. W. et al. Countercurrent immunoelectrophoresis in group B streptococcal disease. *Pediatrics* 64:632–634, 1979.

4. Typlin, B. L. et al. Counter immunoelectrophoresis for the rapid diagnosis of group B streptococcal infections. *Clin. Pediatr.* 18:366–369, 1979.

5. Ward, J. I. et al. Rapid diagnosis of hemophilus influenzae type b infections by latex particle agglutination and counter immunoelectrophoresis. *J. Pediatr.* 93:37–42, 1978.

6. Marks, M. I., and Welch, D. F. Diagnosis of bacterial infections of the newborn infant. *Clin. Perinatol.* 8:537–558, 1981.

7. Baker, C. J. et al. Countercurrent immunoelectrophoresis in the evaluation of infants with group B streptococcal disease. *Pediatrics* 65:1110–1114, 1980.

8. Edwards, M. S.; Kasper, D. L.; and Baker, C. J. Rapid diagnosis of type III group B streptococcal meningitis by latex particle agglutination. *J. Pediatr.* 95:202–205, 1979.

9. Bromberger, P. I. et al. Rapid detection of neonatal group B streptococcal infections by latex agglutination. *J. Pediatr.* 96:104–106, 1980.

10. Ingram, D. L. et al. Group B streptococcal disease: its diagnosis with the use of antigen detection, Gram's stain and the presence of apnea and hypotension. *Am. J. Dis. Child.* 134:754–758, 1980.

11. Kumar, A., and Nankervis, G. A. Latex agglutination test and countercurrent immunoelectrophoresis for detection of group B streptococcal antigen. *J. Pediatr.* 96:786–787, 1980.

12. Scheifele, D. W.; Ward, J. I; and Siber, G. R. Advantage of latex agglutination over countercurrent immunoelectrophoresis in the detection of *Haemophilus influenzae* type b antigen in serum. *Pediatrics* 68:888–891, 1981.

13. Kaplan, S. L., and Feigin, R. D. Rapid identification of the invading organism. *Pediatr. Clin. North Am.* 27:783–803, 1980.

14. Polin, R. A., and Kennett, R. Use of monoclonal antibodies in an enzyme-linked inhibition assay for rapid detection of streptococcal antigen. *J. Pediatr.* 97:540–544, 1980.

15. Morrow, D. L. et al. Rapid detection of group B streptococcal antigen by monoclonal antibody sandwich enzyme assay (abstr.). *Pediatr. Res.* 17:278A, 1983.

16. Yolken, R. H., and Hughes, W. I. Rapid diagnosis of infections caused by β-lactamase-producing bacteria by means of an enzyme radioisotopic assay. *J. Pediatr.* 97:715–720, 1980.

17. Ryan, M. E., and Barrett, F. Rapid detection of group B streptococcal colonization by a direct immunofluorescent antibody technique. *J. Pediatr.* 101:993–995, 1982.

18. Rom, S.; Flynn, D.; and Noone, P. Anaerobic infection in a neonate: early detection by gas liquid chromatography and response to metranidazole. *Arch. Dis. Child.* 52:740–741, 1977.

19. Laforce, F. M.; Brice, J. L.; and Tornabene, T. G. Diagnosis of bacterial meningitis by gas-liquid chromatography. II: Analysis of spinal fluid. *J. Infect. Dis.* 140:453–464, 1979.

20. Kleiman, M. B. et al. Acridine orange stain for body fluid examination (abstr.). *Pediatr. Res.* 17:273A, 1983.

ELEVEN

Management

Antimicrobial Treatment

Antibiotics undoubtedly are the mainstay of treatment of neonatal sepsis and meningitis; however, it may be more correct to talk about antimicrobial agents, as the first advance in treatment was the introduction of sulfonamides in the late thirties. At present, the resurgence of many different bacteria that are resistant to commonly employed antibiotics means that other antimicrobials are being evaluated.

Perhaps the simplest way of looking at antibiotic therapy is to say that—where practicable—antibiotics should be used for as short a period as possible and that local sensitivities of various bacteria should be incorporated into the choice of specific antibiotic(s). Nevertheless, as emphasized elsewhere,[1] "a disturbingly prevalent attitude is that antibiotics can do little harm. This, of course, is not true." When antibiotics *are* started, "every effort should be made to discontinue their use at the earliest possible time."[2] This is usually possible within 48 to 72 hours, when culture results are negative.[1,2]

In dealing with neonatal sepsis and meningitis, certain assumptions have to be made, because it is not possible to wait for the results of cultures. The rapidity of deterioration in neonates with sepsis can be quite dramatic, with death occurring within a few hours. Consequently, the most appropriate antibiotics for the most likely bacterial organisms must be chosen (see table 11.1). As indicated in chapter 2, the most

Table 11.1.

Common Drugs Used to Treat Sepsis and Meningitis: First Week-Antibiotic Treatment*

Antibiotic	Usual dose (kg/day, q 12 hr)	Route	Effective against	Minimum inhibitory concentration (µg/ml)	Achievable serum concentration dose (µg/ml)
Penicillin G	50,000–100,000 units	IV, IM	‡GBS	<0.1	36–60
			§GDS	3.1	
			Listeria	0.8	
			monocytogenes		
			? E. coli	50	
			? Proteus	25	
			(indole −)		
Ampicillin	100–200 mg	IV, IM	GBS	<0.1	180–200
			GDS	1.6	
			Listeria	0.4	
			E. coli	3.1	
			? Klebsiella	50	
			pneumoniae		
			? Proteus	50	
			(indole −)		
Gentamicin	5 mg†	IV, IM	S. aureus	3.1	2–8
			Listeria	3.1	
			E. coli	3.1	
			K. pneumoniae	0.4	
			Proteus (indole +)	0.4	
			? Pseudomonas	6.3	

Antibiotic	Dose	Route	Organism		
Nafcillin	50–100 mg	IV, IM	GBS	<0.1	22–70
			S. aureus	0.4	
			?GDS	12.5	
			?Listeria	6.3	
Chloramphenicol	25 mg	IV	?GBS	6.3	14–27
			?E. coli	6.3	
			?K. pneumoniae	6.3	
			?Proteus (indole +)	6.3	
Moxalactam	50–100 mg	IV	?GBS	6.3	70–210
			?S. aureus	12.5	
			E. coli	<0.1	
			K. pneumoniae	0.2	
			Proteus (indole + and −)	<0.1	
Cefotaxime	50–100 mg	IV	GBS	<0.1	26–52
			S. aureus	1.6	
			E. coli	<0.1	
			K. pneumoniae	<0.1	
			Proteus (indole + and −)	<0.1	

Modified from B. Dashefsky and J. O. Klein. The treatment of bacterial infections in the newborn infant. *Clin. Perinatol.* 8:559–577, 1981.

*In general, dose/day remains constant, but frequency of administration increases to q 8 hr after the first week.

†May need to reduce to 2.5 mg q 24 hr in infants <1500 g.

‡GBS = group B streptococci.

§GDS = group D streptococci.

common organisms currently encountered in the first 5 to 7 days after birth are still *Escherichia coli* and group B streptococci (GBS), for the majority of the United States and Canada. In certain parts of the country and in other countries, however, quite different organisms may predominate.[3-6] Nevertheless, assuming that *E. coli* and GBS are the most prevalent organisms, the treatment of choice usually will be the combination of a penicillin and an aminoglycoside.[7-10] The penicillin used usually is aqueous penicillin G, which may be most useful for GBS, or ampicillin, which has the advantage of being effective for both GBS and many strains of *E. coli*. The aminoglycoside of choice is frequently kanamycin, but has been replaced by gentamicin in many centers because of an increase in the number of organisms that are resistant to kanamycin. On the other hand, it cannot be assumed that gentamicin will always be useful, because resistance can develop relatively quickly.[1,11,12] In particular, the nonspecific topical application of gentamicin ointment can lead to acquisition of multiply resistant *Staphylococcus aureus*.[13] (For complications of antibiotics, see chapter 12.)

In addition to the need for more than one antibiotic on the basis of more than one likely prevalent organism, there may be the advantage of synergism between penicillins and aminoglycosides (with a greater effect of the combination than either alone would indicate). Although there are really no clinical data to indicate that survival has been increased by synergism, theoretical advantages have been proposed based on in vitro studies and experimental infections.[14] Ampicillin may be more synergistic than penicillin and, in the context of synergism, carbenicillin is particularly useful with some aminoglycosides (but not kanamycin) in the treatment of *Pseudomonas* infection.[8,14]

After the first 4 days or so, there is an increasing possibility that infection will be caused by *S. aureus* or to an organism associated with the equipment surrounding the baby, such as *Pseudomonas aeruginosa, Serratia marcescens,* or other "water bugs." Because of this likelihood, from the end of the first week onward, it may be preferable to start antimicrobial treatment with a penicillinase-resistant penicillin and an aminoglycoside other than kanamycin.[10,14] In a study in infants and children, nafcillin was less likely than methicillin to be associated with urologic toxicity; therefore, if the organism is sensitive to both, nafcillin may offer a theoretical advantage.[15]

Approach to Antibiotic Treatment

As noted earlier, the diversity of clinical manifestations that can indicate sepsis results in a large number of infants being treated without culture evidence of infection. Under many circumstances, it is difficult to know how to manage the neonate without using antibiotics; however, this difficulty may result in many babies being treated unnecessarily. For example, when two Boston hospitals were compared, the ratio of infants treated with antibiotics to those with proved sepsis was 15:1 in one hospital and 28:1 in the other.[16] In the author's experience, it was possible to incorporate several simple diagnostic tests into antibiotic decisions and decrease the ratio from 11:1 to 6.6:1.[17] With even greater selection, the ratio possibly could be decreased even further (e.g., 5:1 or 4:1), but this will depend a good deal on the characteristics of the neonatal population being investigated.

Although elaborate flow diagrams for decision-making can be designed, it may be simpler to think of factors that either favor or oppose the use of antibiotics. Clinical skill in evaluating the individual baby undoubtedly is an important part of thoughtful antibiotic administration because, unfortunately, it is too easy to treat everybody for the least indication. Too, not enough attention has been directed toward evaluating what features influence the seasoned clinician to believe that a baby has sepsis. In one recent study the following findings were strongly associated with neonatal infection: tachycardia or arrhythmia, decreased peripheral perfusion, pallor, irritability, abdominal distention, apnea, hypo- or hypertension, and lethargy.[18] In another study skin discoloration, poor perfusion, hypotonia, bradycardia, apnea, hepatomegaly and gastrointestinal tract signs were considered the most helpful features for early diagnosis.[19] Both studies also included hematologic findings in their attempts to make an early diagnosis (see also chapter 8).

The following factors favor the use of antibiotics:

1. Preterm infant
2. Multiple risk factors suggesting exposure to infection
3. Clinical signs suggesting infection (see Appendix tables 2 and 3 for the yield from individual signs)

4. Positive diagnostic tests (e.g., abnormal leukocyte count, increased C-reactive protein, or CRP, levels; see chapter 8)

The following factors oppose but do not negate the use of antibiotics:

1. Term infant
2. Single risk factor
3. Absence of clinical signs (i.e., "asymptomatic")
4. Negative diagnostic tests (see chapter 8)

In those infants for whom a decision not to use antibiotics has been made, careful reappraisal 8 to 12 hours later should be mandatory. When antibiotics *are* initiated, reevaluation at 48 to 72 hours is required to decide whether or not antibiotics can be stopped at that time. This time frame is chosen because 96% to 98% of blood cultures become positive within 48 to 72 hours.[2]

Another major consideration is the age of the baby at the time of evaluation—although it should be apparent that risk factors are only applicable in the 48 hours or so immediately after birth. The decision to use or not use antibiotics is a little simpler in the neonate being evaluated for risk factors. It is more difficult when clinical signs point toward infection, particularly after the first week following delivery. For instance, the development of jaundice or apnea on the third or fourth day is unlikely to be due to sepsis (although it can be), whereas the sudden onset of jaundice or apnea at 2 weeks of age would be much more suggestive of sepsis.

As stated earlier, during the first 4 days, ampicillin and kanamycin seem to be appropriate starting therapy although gentamicin frequently is used instead of kanamycin. One recent study showed that the sensitivity of *E. coli* and *Klebsiella* to kanamycin and gentamicin was rarely different.[20] After 4 days, gentamicin and methicillin (or oxacillin or nafcillin) might be more appropriate therapy, particularly for the infant requiring assisted ventilation. When staphylococci are known to be resistant to methicillin, vancomycin may also be a first-choice antibiotic.[21,22]

In cases of meningitis, the most important consideration is that the antibiotic chosen will penetrate into cerebrospinal fluid. For this reason, although ampicillin may still be valuable (especially against gram-positive organisms), chloramphenicol remains a very useful drug against gram-negative organisms, provided that care is taken to use the correct dose at the start of treatment and to follow serum levels at intervals.[23,24] In addition, the third-generation cephalosporins, such as moxalactam and cefotaxime, have been used increasingly in the neonatal period against gram-negative organisms[9,10,25,26] and are also effective against GBS and *S. aureus* (cefotaxime is superior to moxalactam against the latter two organisms).

Because the duration of antibiotics currently is rather empirical, it is usually advised that in cases of sepsis, antibiotics should be given for 7 to 10 days and in cases of meningitis for 14 to 21 days, depending on the organism. Objective data on which to base such decisions are lacking. It is possible that sequential measurements of levels of acute-phase reactants (such as CRP) could provide the most reliable means of deciding when to stop antibiotics. This approach has recently been supported by the work of Squire and colleagues[27] and Speer and co-workers,[28] which provide some confirmation for the findings of Sabel and Hanson.[29] These latter investigators observed relapses in three cases of meningitis when elevated levels of CRP were noted at the end of antibiotic treatment. In cases where CRP levels had returned to normal before discontinuing antibiotics, no relapses occurred. Thus, CRP levels could be used to indicate when inflammation has subsided and several extra days of antibiotics (e.g., 3–4 days) could be given to be safe. Other acute-phase reactants (e.g., α_1-acid glycoprotein) appear to subside more slowly and could provide additional supportive evidence that the infection has been controlled. With this scheme, a decline in levels of CRP after 3 or 4 days is likely with uncomplicated sepsis, while approximately 1 week or more is needed for α_1-acid glycoprotein to return to normal (fig. 11.1). In some cases of meningitis, the length of time for the acute-phase reactants to return to normal is more protracted, which is in agreement with current policies regarding antibiotic therapy. After 3–4 days, levels can be measured every 2–3 days.

General Management

Management of the neonate with sepsis is directed toward allowing this immunocompromised host to combat bacterial invasion of the blood-

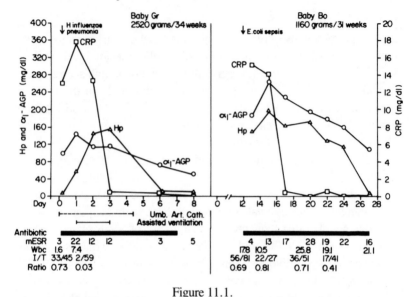

Figure 11.1.

*Quantitative determinations of C-reactive protein (CRP), haptoglobin (Hp),
and α_1-acid glycoprotein (α_1-AGP) levels in infants with* Haemophilus
influenzae *pneumonia and* Escherichia coli *sepsis are contrasted with
leukocyte and ESR values. I/T = immature to total neutrophil ratio.*

stream. In addition to antibiotic therapy directed at specific organisms,
it is also important to support the baby, both in ways that minimize
derangement of homeostasis and in ways that may contribute to combating infection. Some of the clinical manifestations clearly demand a
specific course of action (e.g., profound apnea will necessitate the use
of assisted ventilation), but there are certain adjunctive measures that
can be taken in almost every case.

Thermoregulation

Maintenance of body temperature is important in all neonates but particularly in those who are preterm and more likely to develop sepsis.
Prevention of cooling (or treating hypothermia if it is present) helps
decrease oxygen demand and minimize any tendency to develop meta-

bolic acidosis. As noted earlier (chap. 5), there may be a decrease in peripheral blood flow secondary to infection, with decreased temperature of the extremities compared with core body temperature.

It is rarely necessary to provide an environmental temperature above the usual neutral thermal environment designated for gestational age or birth weight and postnatal age. Nevertheless, it is important that the neutral thermal environment is provided, to decrease cold stress. It is also helpful to use intravenous glucose (i.e., dextrose) to provide a reliable source of glucose, which can be metabolized aerobically to produce heat.

Oxygen

It is usually necessary to provide supplemental oxygen to septic neonates, although their needs will vary depending on the severity of the illness. In preterm infants, oxygen administration must be monitored carefully to keep PaO_2 levels within normal limits, to minimize the potential toxicity to the eye (i.e., retrolental fibroplasia or retinopathy of prematurity).

Adequate oxygenation is important for several reasons. Oxygen is needed for heat production (see Thermoregulation). Respiratory distress, one of the more common manifestations of sepsis, can be caused by associated pneumonia or can be secondary to persistent pulmonary hypertension; assisted ventilation using an endotracheal tube and respirator may be needed to maintain adequate oxygenation. Adequate oxygenation will decrease any tendency toward metabolic acidosis, thereby decreasing the peripheral vasoconstriction that may accompany sepsis, which is presumably secondary to endotoxin or endotoxinlike products released by bacteria.

Blood Products

There are two major reasons for administering blood products in neonatal sepsis: (1) to combat shock and (2) to provide factors that may be deficient in host defense.

Simple Transfusion

The most usual method of combating shock is to provide additional fluid in the form of fresh-frozen plasma or whole blood (either fresh or reconstituted), although any fluid may be appropriate in an emergency. In addition, fresh-frozen plasma or whole blood will provide opsonic factors (presumably complement as well as antibody) that aid phago-cytosis.[30] There may also be sufficient transfer of specific antibody to be effective in decreasing mortality with certain bacteria (e.g., GBS).[31,32]

Exchange Transfusion

Exchange transfusion has been used by a number of investigators, usu-ally in the presence of such severe manifestations of sepsis as sclerema (see chapter 5).[33-38] In addition to the benefits conferred by simple transfusion, with transfer of antibody more likely to be effective, there may also be removal of circulating bacteria and endotoxin.[38] Several authors have concluded that exchange transfusion has saved infants with sepsis who would otherwise have died,[33-37] however, the evi-dence is not conclusive at this time, as most studies were not controlled trials.

Granulocyte Transfusion

Another adjunct to therapy arises from the demonstration that many infants with overwhelming sepsis have profound neutropenia (see chapter 8). The work of Christensen and Rothstein has shown that when neutrophil counts are low and are associated with very high im-mature/total neutrophil ratios, the neutrophil storage pool in the bone marrow can be severely depleted.[39] Because of this, they as well as others have used granulocyte transfusions under these circumstances, with apparently dramatic success in decreasing mortality[40,41]; however, the evidence is based on comparatively small numbers at this time. There is also a considerable time lag in being able to make such a trans-fusion available, because fresh blood is required and cells need to be irradiated before administration. Consequently, in those cases where the need is greatest, the time interval from the decision to treat to receipt of granulocytes for transfusion may preclude effective therapy. Nevertheless, this technique does seem to be an important adjunct to therapy in some cases.[42]

Hyperventilation

Many infants with neonatal sepsis and meningitis require assisted ventilation to treat respiratory distress, apnea, or coma. Hyperventilation may be useful in two specific circumstances: (1) in the presence of persistent pulmonary hypertension (i.e., persistent fetal circulation), when lowering PCO_2 and increasing pH to produce alkalemia may enhance pulmonary perfusion[43]; and (2) when increased intracranial pressure is suspected or documented in cases of meningitis.[44,45] Hyperventilation can decrease cerebral blood flow, which may be advantageous in decreasing intracranial pressure, but could be deleterious when carried to extremes.

Sodium Bicarbonate

As noted earlier, poor peripheral perfusion and shock may result in metabolic acidosis. Many neonates will spontaneously hyperventilate by becoming tachypneic and blowing off carbon dioxide to compensate for such acidosis, but in many cases it is necessary to minimize the stress placed on the baby by giving bicarbonate. In an emergency, 2 mEq/kg sodium bicarbonate can be given by slow push.

Miscellaneous Factors

In most cases where infants are sick enough to be placed in an intensive care nursery, management with heart rate, respiration, and blood pressure monitoring will be routine. In addition, most babies can be managed with continuous transcutaneous PO_2 measurements, particularly when persistent pulmonary hypertension is suspected. In babies with meningitis, it can also be advantageous to use continuous intracranial pressure monitoring, using a noninvasive device (such as the Ladd sensor) placed over the anterior fontanelle.[45,46] It may also be advisable to limit fluid intake somewhat, until adequate urine output has been demonstrated. This factor is particularly important in infants who appear edematous, as the syndrome of inappropriate antidiuretic hormone secretion (SIADH) has been described in infants with meningitis.[47,48] Treatment of SIADH is by restricting fluid intake.

The use of anti-inflammatory drugs has not been well studied in the neonate, but corticosteroids are not believed to confer any advantage. Recent animal data suggest that nonsteroidal anti-inflammatory agents such as indomethacin might be beneficial, but probably would need to be given very shortly after infection was acquired, which suggests that they may be impractical.[49] Following reports of its use in adults, naloxone has also been used in neonates with septic shock, with apparent benefit.[50] Infants were given 10 to 15 µg/kg naloxone as a loading dose, followed by a continuous infusion of 10 to 15 µg/kg/hr for at least 24 hours.[50]

Prophylaxis

Because of the increased susceptibility of neonates to infection, it seems desirable to try to prevent the acquisition of virulent organisms or to increase the defense mechanisms of the neonate. Two approaches have been adopted, but each has its drawbacks, although the advantages may outweigh the disadvantages under certain circumstances.

Immunoprophylaxis

The general approach of immunoprophylaxis is to take advantage of the fact that immunoglobulin G is transferred from mother to baby across the placenta. If the mother can be induced to produce antibody to the most likely neonatal pathogens, the baby could be protected. For instance, it is well established that infants who acquire early-onset GBS infection have mothers who lack antibody to the specific type of GBS causing infection.[51,52] If GBS infection is prevalent, it would be useful to use a polyvalent vaccine to induce antibody in the mother during pregnancy. At present, there is a vaccine available for type III GBS that is immunogenic and potentially useful; however, it does not provide protection against the other types, which account for 40% to 50% of neonatal GBS sepsis. Research continues in this area to answer questions about effectiveness and cost-benefit ratios.[53]

One of the problems with the vaccine approach is that prevalent organisms change with the passage of time. Another major pathogen, *E. coli,* does not lend itself readily to immunoprophylaxis, partly because there are so many serotypes, but also because the major antibody response is in the immunoglobulin M fraction, which does not cross the placenta. At other times, or in other countries, there may not be an available vaccine for use against the most prevalent organisms.

For these reasons, it is unlikely that immunoprophylaxis will have widespread application, except perhaps in certain high-risk situations when preterm delivery is anticipated or a given organism is particularly prevalent. In the case of preterm delivery, the fact that maternal antibody transfer seems to be deficient prior to 34 weeks' gestation may severely limit the usefulness of this approach.

Chemoprophylaxis

Just as immunoprophylaxis has been directed primarily toward GBS infection, so too has chemoprophylaxis.[53] The principal approach arose from the observation that in one New York hospital where a single dose of penicillin was administered soon after birth to prevent gonococcal ophthalmia early-onset GBS infection was not seen in the neonates, despite the fact that most other hospitals in North America were encountering the organism quite frequently.[54] Subsequently a large-scale controlled trial was conducted in Dallas, alternating penicillin injection with topical tetracycline on a monthly basis. A decrease in the incidence and mortality of GBS sepsis was confirmed[55,56]; however, there was an increase initially in the incidence of gram-negative organisms, which can produce more difficulty in treatment.[55] In contrast to these findings, experience in Chicago was quite the opposite. No decrease in incidence or mortality was observed with a randomized controlled trial in low birth weight infants.[57] Whether the focus on low birth weight infants accounts for the difference seems unlikely, although the Chicago group have also demonstrated that high mortality is associated with very low birth weight.[58]

In summary, the conflicting results suggest that in the group with the highest mortality risk there is little benefit to administering a single dose of penicillin soon after birth. In term infants (with lower mortality), there may be some benefit in preventing early-onset infection, but there does not appear to be a diminution in the incidence of late-onset infection.

The other chemoprophylactic approach is to try to identify the mother who is carrying GBS and to treat the mother prior to delivery. The most effective way to do this seems to be with the intrapartum administration of ampicillin or penicillin.[59,60] There seems to be agreement that attempting to eradicate GBS earlier in pregnancy results in only temporary absence of colonization.[61] It is also apparent that the ratio of treated mothers to infected—not just colonized—babies is approximately 50:1 to 100:1.[62,63] By selectively culturing only women who have preterm labor or premature rupture of membranes, it may be possible to decrease the ratio to 20:1.[64] Whether or not such an approach is cost effective remains somewhat debatable, but intrapartum screening seems preferable to antepartum screening.[65]

Apart from extensive investigations concerning GBS, there is little information about attempts to prevent neonatal sepsis caused by other organisms. There is a tendency for obstetricians to withhold treatment of the mother suspected of having chorioamnionitis, because pediatricians have thought that this would confuse interpretation in the neonate. It seems more logical to treat the mother, however, in order to prevent the neonate from being infected. Under these circumstances, cultures can be sent and antibiotics started on the baby. If cultures are negative in the baby and there is no evidence of infection using leukocyte counts and acute-phase protein level determinations, antibiotics could be stopped after 48 to 72 hours. If acute-phase proteins are elevated or antigen is demonstrated in body fluids (by countercurrent immunoelectrophoresis or latex particle agglutination test), it would be advisable to treat for 7 days.

References

1. Prober, C. G., and Gold, R. Antibiotic abuse: spare the child. *Can. Med. Assoc. J.* 122:7–8, 1980.

2. Pichichero, M. E., and Todd, J. K. Detection of neonatal bacteremia. *J. Pediatr.* 94:958–965, 1979.

3. Tafari, N., and Ljungh-Wadstrom, A. Consequences of amniotic fluid infection: early neonatal septicemia. In *Perinatal infections.* Ciba Foundation Symposium, No. 77. New York: Elsevier-North Holland, 1980, pp. 55–62.

4. Bennet, R.; Eriksson, M.; and Zetterström, R. Increasing incidence of neonatal septicemia: causative organisms and predisposing risk factors. *Acta Paediatr. Scand.* 70:207–210, 1981.

5. Ohlsson, A., and Serenius, F. Neonatal septicemia in Riyadh, Saudi Arabia. *Acta Paediatr. Scand.* 70:825–829, 1981.

6. Placzek, M. M., and Whitelaw, A. Early and late neonatal septicemia. *Arch. Dis. Child.* 58:728–731, 1983.

7. McCracken, G. H., Jr. Pharmacologic basis for antimicrobial therapy in newborn infants. *Am. J. Dis. Child.* 28:407–419, 1974.

8. Dashefsky, B., and Klein, J. O. The treatment of bacterial infections in the newborn infant. *Clin. Perinatol.* 8:559–577, 1981.

9. Harris, M. C., and Polin, R. A. Neonatal septicemia. *Pediatr. Clin. North Am.* 30:243–258, 1983.

10. Klein, J. O. et al. Selection of antimicrobial agents for treatment of neonatal sepsis. *Rev. Infect. Dis.* 5(Suppl.):S55–S62, 1983.

11. Grylack, L. J., and Scanlon, J. W. Oral gentamicin therapy in the prevention of neonatal necrotizing enterocolitis. *Am. J. Dis. Child.* 132:1192–1194, 1978.

12. Franco, J. A.; Eitzman, D. V.; and Baer, H. Antibiotic usage and microbial resistance in an intensive care nursery. *Am. J. Dis. Child.* 126:318–321, 1973.

13. Graham, D. R. et al. Epidemic neonatal gentamicin-methicillin-resistant *Staphylococcus aureus* infection associated with non-specific topical use of gentamicin. *J. Pediatr.* 97:972–978, 1980.

14. Bell, W. E., and McGuiness, G. A. Suppurative central nervous system infections in the neonate. *Semin. Perinatol.* 6:1–24, 1982.

15. Kitzing, W.; Nelson, J. D.; and Mohs, E. Comparative toxicities of methicillin and nafcillin. *Am. J. Dis. Child.* 135:52–55, 1981.

16. Hammerschlag, M. R. et al. Patterns of use of antibiotics in two newborn nurseries. *N. Engl. J. Med.* 296:1268–1269, 1977.

17. Philip, A. G. S. Decreased use of antibiotics using a neonatal sepsis screening technique. *J. Pediatr.* 98:795–799, 1981.

18. Spector, S. A.; Ticknor, W.; and Grossman, M. Study of the usefulness of clinical and hematologic findings in the diagnosis of neonatal bacterial infections. *Clin. Pediatr.* 20:385–392, 1981.

19. Töllner, U. Early diagnosis of septicemia in the newborn: clinical studies and sepsis score. *Eur. J. Pediatr.* 138:331–337, 1982.

20. Grylack, L.; Neugebauer, D.; and Scanlon, J. W. Effects of oral antibiotics on stool flora and overall sensitivity patterns in an intensive care nursery. *Pediatr. Res.* 16:509–511, 1982.

21. Schaad, U. B. et al. Clinical pharmacology and efficacy of vancomycin in pediatric patients. *J. Pediatr.* 96:119–126, 1980.

22. Baumgart, S. et al. Sepsis with coagulase-negative staphylococci in critically ill newborns. *Am. J. Dis. Child.* 137:461–463, 1983.

23. Rajchgot, P. et al. Initiation of chloramphenicol therapy in the newborn infant. *J. Pediatr.* 101:1018–1021, 1982.

24. Mulhall, A.; De Louvois, J.; and Hurley, R. Efficacy of chloramphenicol in the treatment of neonatal and infantile meningitis: a study of 70 cases. *Lancet* 1:284–287, 1983.

25. Schaad, U. B. et al. Clinical evaluation of a new broad-spectrum oxa-beta-lactam antibiotic, moxalactam, in neonates and infants. *J. Pediatr.* 98:129–136, 1981.

26. Kafetzis, D. A. et al. Treatment of severe neonatal infections with cefotaxime: efficacy and pharmacokinetics. *J. Pediatr.* 100:483–489, 1982.

27. Squire, E. N., Jr. et al. Criteria for the discontinuation of antibiotic therapy during presumptive treatment of suspected neonatal infection. *Pediatr. Infect. Dis.* 1:85–90, 1982.

28. Speer, C.; Bruns, A.; and Gahr, M. Sequential determination of CRP, α_1-antitrypsin and haptoglobin in neonatal septicemia. *Acta Paediatr. Scand.* 72:679–683, 1983.

29. Sabel, K. G., and Hanson, L. A. The clinical usefulness of C-reactive protein (CRP) determinations in bacterial meningitis and septicemia in infancy. *Acta Paediatr. Scand.* 63:381–388, 1974.

30. Bortolussi, R.; Issekutz, A. C.; and Barnard, D. R. The use of plasma infusion for neonatal sepsis (abstr.). *Pediatr. Res.* 15:607, 1981.

31. Courtney, S. E.; Hall, R. T.; and Harris, D. J. Effect of blood-transfusions on mortality in early-onset group B streptococcal septicaemia. *Lancet* 2:462–463, 1979.

32. Hall, R. T. et al. Effect of blood transfusions on group B streptococcal antibody levels (abstr.). *Pediatr. Res.* 15:613, 1981.

33. Xanthou, M. et al. Exchange transfusion in severe neonatal infection with sclerema. *Arch. Dis. Child.* 50:901–902, 1975.

34. Töllner, U. et al. Treatment of septicaemia in the newborn infant: choice of initial antimicrobial drugs and the role of exchange transfusion. *Acta Paediatr. Scand.* 66:605–610, 1977.

35. Belohdrasky, B. H.; Roos, R.; and Marget, W. Exchange transfusion in neonatal septicemia. *Infection* 6:S139, 1978.

36. Pelet, B. Exchange transfusion in newborn infants: effects on granulocyte function. *Arch. Dis. Child.* 54:687–690, 1979.

37. Vain, N. E. et al. Role of exchange transfusion in the treatment of severe septicemia. *Pediatrics* 66:693–697, 1980.

38. Togari, H. et al. Endotoxin clearance by exchange blood transfusion in septic shock neonates. *Acta Paediatr. Scand.* 72:87–91, 1983.

39. Christensen, R. D., and Rothstein, G. Exhaustion of mature marrow neutrophils in neonates with sepsis. *J. Pediatr.* 96:316–318, 1980.

40. Laurenti, F. et al. Polymorphonuclear leukocyte transfusion for the treatment of sepsis in the newborn infant. *J. Pediatr.* 98:118–123, 1981.

41. Christensen, R. D. et al. Granulocyte transfusions in neonates with bacterial infection, neutropenia, and depletion of mature marrow neutrophils. *Pediatrics* 70:1–6, 1982.

42. Hill, H. R. Phagocyte transfusion—ultimate therapy of neonatal disease? *J. Pediatr.* 98:59–61, 1981.

43. Drummond, W. H. et al. The independent effects of hyperventilation, tolazoline, and dopamine on infants with persistent pulmonary hypertension. *J. Pediatr.* 98:603–611, 1981.

44. Goitein, K. J.; Amit, Y.; and Mussaffi, H. Intracranial pressure in central nervous system infections and cerebral ischaemia of infancy. *Arch. Dis. Child.* 58:184–186, 1983.

45. McMenamin, J. B., and Volpe, J. J. Bacterial meningitis in infants: effects on intracranial pressure (ICP) and cerebral blood flow (CBF) velocity (abstr.). *Pediatr. Res.* 17:284A, 1983.

46. Philip, A. G. S. Non-invasive monitoring of intracranial pressure: a new approach for neonatal clinical pharmacology. *Clin. Perinatol.* 6:123–137, 1979.

47. Gotoff, S. P., and Behrman, R. E. Neonatal septicemia. *J. Pediatr.* 76:142–153, 1970.

48. Feigin, R. D. et al. Inappropriate secretion of antidiuretic hormone (ADH) in children with bacterial meningitis. *Am. J. Clin. Nutr.* 30:1482–1484, 1977.

49. Short, B. L.; Miller, M. K.; and Fletcher, J. R. Improved survival in the suckling rat model of group B streptococcal sepsis after treatment with non-steroidal anti-inflammatory drugs. *Pediatrics* 70:343–347, 1982.

50. Eriksson, M. Neonatal septicemia. *Acta Paediatr. Scand.* 72:1–8, 1983.

51. Vogel, L. C. et al. Prevalence of type-specific group B streptococcal antibody in pregnant women. *J. Pediatr.* 96:1047–1051, 1980.

52. Baker, C. J.; Edwards, M. S.; and Kasper, D. L. Role of antibody to native type III polysaccharide of group B streptococcus in infant infection. *Pediatrics* 68:544–549, 1981.

53. Interview with Carol J. Baker, M.D. Prevention of neonatal group B streptococcal disease. *Pediatr. Infect. Dis.* 2:1–6, 1983.

54. Steigman, A. J.; Bottone, E. J.; and Hanna, B. A. Intramuscular penicillin administration at birth: prevention of early-onset group B streptococcal disease. *Pediatrics* 62:842–844, 1978.

55. Siegel, J. D. et al. Single-dose penicillin prophylaxis against neonatal group B streptococcal infection: a controlled trial in 18,730 newborn infants. *N. Engl. J. Med.* 303:769–775, 1980.

56. Siegel, J. D. et al. Single-dose penicillin prophylaxis in neonatal group B streptococcal disease: conclusion of a 41 month controlled trial. *Lancet* 1:1426–1430, 1982.

57. Pyati, S. P. et al. Penicillin in infants weighing two kilograms or less with early-onset group B streptococcal disease. *N. Engl. J. Med.* 308:1383–1388, 1983.

58. Pyati, S. P. et al. Decreasing mortality in neonates with early-onset group B streptococcal infection: reality or artifact? *J. Pediatr.* 98:625–627, 1981.

59. Yow, M. D. et al. Ampicillin prevents intrapartum transmission of group B streptococcus. *J.A.M.A.* 241:1245–1247, 1979.

60. Easmon, C. S. F. et al. The effect of intrapartum chemoprophylaxis on the vertical transmission of group B streptococci. *Br. J. Obstet. Gynaecol.* 90:633–635, 1983.

61. Gardner, S. E. et al. Failure of penicillin to eradicate group B streptococcal colonization in the pregnant woman couple study. *Am. J. Obstet. Gynecol.* 135:1062–1065, 1979.

62. Davis, J. P. et al. Vertical transmission of group B streptococcus. *J.A.M.A.* 242:42–44, 1979.

63. Baker, C. J. Group B streptococcal infections in neonates. *Pediatrics in Review* 1:5–15, 1979.

64. Pasnick, M.; Mead, P. B.; and Philip, A. G. S. Selective maternal culturing to identify group B streptococcal infection. *Am. J. Obstet. Gynecol.* 138:480–484, 1980.

65. Iams, J. D., and O'Shaughnessy, R. Antepartum versus intrapartum selective screening for maternal group B streptococcal colonization. *Am. J. Obstet. Gynecol.* 143:153–156, 1982.

T W E L V E

Prognosis

Mortality

As mentioned in the introduction, mortality from neonatal sepsis in the preantibiotic era was greater than 90%, which accounts for the discrepancy between the frequency with which antimicrobials are used and the actual documentation of systemic bacterial infection. Because the presentation can be so subtle and many babies die so rapidly, the clinician is fearful of missing a diagnosis that is susceptible to treatment.

Despite the aggressive approach to detection and treatment of neonatal sepsis that is adopted in most neonatal intensive care units, the mortality remains disturbingly high at approximately 25%.[1-4] Often forgotten in this generalization is the fact that infants of low birth weight are particularly susceptible and may have an increasing risk as birth weight—and gestational age—decreases. In 1965, Buetow and colleagues documented an overall rate of sepsis of 54 per 1000 live births considered premature (i.e., low birth weight). The respective rates for babies with birth weights 1001 to 1500 g, 1501 to 2000 g, and 2001 to 2500 g were 164, 91, and 23 per 1000 live births.[5] Mortality in septicemic infants was 50%, in contrast to 6.6% in the nonsepticemic group.[5]

In my Vermont series, the overall mortality of infants with sepsis was 24% (10 of 41 infants died); however, 9 of 24 low birth weight infants died, while only 1 of 17 infants with birth weight ≥ 2500 g died. This has been emphasized by Pyati and colleagues in Chicago.[6]

They documented that an apparent improvement in survival of neonates with early-onset group B streptococcal (GBS) infection was entirely due to a shift in the birth weight distribution of infected infants. The death rate in infants of very low birth weight ($<$ 1500 g) was almost 100%, whereas those of normal birth weight ($\geq$ 2500 g) had a rate of 20% to 25%.[6] Particularly with regard to GBS infection, the age at onset or detection of sepsis seems to be very important. Mortality is particularly high when sepsis is documented within 24 hours of delivery (see chapter 2).[4,7] This high mortality may be because many infants are infected in utero and do not receive appropriate antibiotic therapy until the infection is well established.

The majority of deaths from sepsis seem to be caused by the effects of shock, with resultant poor cardiac output, poor perfusion, increasing metabolic acidosis, and multiple organ dysfunction. In other cases, intrapartum asphyxia, with or without associated thrombocytopenia or disseminated intravascular coagulation (DIC), can lead to a generalized bleeding tendency, which may include intracranial hemorrhage. Other cases of sepsis may go undetected unless postmortem cultures are obtained, so that the scope of this problem may be underestimated.[8]

Complications

The major complications related to the infectious process itself have been discussed as distant effects in chapter 6. These complications include persistent pulmonary hypertension, cholestatic jaundice, disorders of glucose metabolism, and electrolyte disturbance. Another comparatively frequent observation is a bleeding tendency. As noted earlier, this may be secondary to an asphyxial insult, to thrombocytopenia, or to DIC. The presence of DIC is documented by decreased platelets, increased prothrombin and partial thromboplastin times, decreased fibrinogen levels, and increased levels of fibrin-split products.[9]

Other complications relate more to the treatment used for the underlying problem. Fluid administration needs to be carefully monitored—particularly in cases of meningitis—because of the tendency to develop the syndrome of inappropriate antidiuretic hormone release. Because asphyxia and shock can also accompany sepsis, there is frequently poor urinary output secondary to decreased glomerular filtration and renal tubular damage. This is usually of short duration when the infection is responsive to therapy; however, urine output should be measured carefully and body weight checked at frequent intervals (2 or 3 times per day) to minimize the tendency to retain fluid. If fluid retention does occur, it is more likely to both impose a strain on already compromised myocardium and increase intracranial pressure.

In those infants who require assisted ventilation, the potential complications of blocked tubes and air leaks (particularly pneumothorax) should be remembered. Blockage of the endotracheal tube is more likely to occur in cases where sepsis is accompanied by pneumonia. Most cases resolve fairly quickly, so that the complication of bronchopulmonary dysplasia is unlikely to occur.

Some of the most important complications are related to the antimicrobial agents used. Although unlikely to be used for neonatal infection today, it should be remembered that long-acting sulfonamides can compete with bilirubin for binding sites on albumin. Such displacement increases the risk of developing bilirubin toxicity.[10,11] Tetracyclines have also been banished from use in young infants because of their effects on growth and their ability to discolor teeth.[10,12,13] Of more practical importance is the fact that the gray-baby syndrome of cardiovascular collapse associated with chloramphenicol is a dose-related phenomenon. If appropriate doses are given (usually 25 mg/kg/day), it is extremely unlikely that toxic levels will be achieved. Despite the fact that this information has been available for more than 20 years,[14] inappropriate doses are still given, with potentially dire consequences.[15,16] Because even the recommended doses give wide variability of serum concentrations, it is important to determine serum levels.[17-19]

The aminoglycosides (e.g., kanamycin, gentamicin, amikacin) are known to produce ototoxicity and nephrotoxicity, but this is unusual unless some compromise of renal function is already present.[10,20] Some authors recommend monitoring serum levels of aminoglycosides because they are also unpredictable[21,22]; however, such testing is not always readily available and consequently may be rather impractical.

Infants with meningitis can have associated ventriculitis.[23-25] This seems to be almost universal in cases of gram-negative infection and attempts have been made to sterilize the cerebrospinal fluid by using either intrathecal or intraventricular antibiotics. Because any one center tends to see comparatively few cases of meningitis, collaborative studies were designed to evaluate the effectiveness of intrathecal and intraventricular aminoglycoside administration.[26,27] The outcome seemed to be worse in the group treated with intraventricular gentamicin, but there are some difficulties in interpretation because of the inclusion of cases of *Salmonella* meningitis.[25] Direct intraventricular administration certainly appears valuable in some cases.[25] It has been postulated that the direct administration may have a sclerosing effect; however, it is also known that hydrocephalus is a naturally occurring complication of neonatal meningitis in a significant percentage of cases, presumably because increased protein levels produce obstruction of normal CSF dynamics.[24] Improved survival may have been at the expense of major neurologic sequelae in survivors.[25,28]

Follow-Up

The information concerning the long-term outcome of infants with sepsis is rather limited.[29] There is more evidence about the follow-up of cases of neonatal meningitis, but even that is comparatively limited in contrast to some other conditions. The limiting factor is that comparatively few survivors emerge from any one center to make valid interpretations possible.

The duration of follow-up may also have important implications, partly because short-term follow-up may emphasize transient neurologic deficit, but also because long-term follow-up is needed to detect disorders of higher cortical function. With these constraints on interpretation, Volpe combined several follow-up studies on group B streptococcal (GBS) meningitis, and showed that 74% of survivors were normal, but 13% had severe neurologic sequelae (e.g., quadriparesis, microcephaly, cortical blindness).[30]

In one study concerned with follow-up of neonatal sepsis, there were 65 survivors among 90 infants with a diagnosis of neonatal septicemia. Two infants subsequently died of unrelated problems, but the remainder were followed for 2.5 to 6.5 years. Fourteen (22% of the survivors) had handicaps possibly related to sepsis. Only six had "uncomplicated" septicemia, while four had meningitis and four had osteomyelitis. Interpretation was further complicated by the fact that 9 of the 14 with a handicap were delivered preterm (28–36 weeks) and had other problems.[31] Thus, "uncomplicated" sepsis probably has a good prognosis in most cases.

In a series of papers published in 1976, it was noted that initial eradication of GBS from either blood or CSF does not mean that relapse may not occur.[32] Penicillins may fail to eradicate GBS from mucous surfaces of young infants, allowing reinfection—usually meningitis.

A brief review of other follow-up studies up to 1978 indicates that most authors had small series, with high mortality and a significant number of permanent sequelae.[31] It has also been suggested that any improvement in survival would probably be accompanied by a similar increase in major neurologic sequelae.[28] While this might be true for meningitis, it seems unlikely for sepsis alone. A favorable prognosis is most likely to occur when diagnosis is made as early as possible and where attention is given to intensive supportive care.

References

1. Crosson, F. J., Jr. et al. Neonatal sepsis at the Johns Hopkins Hospital. 1969–1975: bacterial isolates and clinical correlates. *Johns Hopkins Med. J.* 140:37–41, 1977.

2. Freedman, R. M. et al. A half century of neonatal sepsis at Yale. *Am. J. Dis. Child.* 135:140–144, 1981.

3. Bennet, R.; Eriksson, M.; and Zetterström, R. Increasing incidence of neonatal septicemia: causative organism and predisposing risk factors. *Acta Paediatr. Scand.* 70:207–210, 1981.

4. Placzek, M. M., and Whitelaw, A. Early and late onset neonatal septicemia. *Arch. Dis. Child.* 58:728–731, 1983.

5. Buetow, K. C.; Klein, S. W.; and Lane, R. B. Septicemia in premature infants. *Am. J. Dis. Child.* 110:29–41, 1965.

6. Pyati, S. P. et al. Decreasing mortality in neonates with early-onset group B streptococcal infection: reality or artifact? *J. Pediatr.* 98:625–627, 1981.

7. Quirante, J.; Ceballos, R.; and Cassady, G. Group B β-hemolytic streptococcal infection in the newborn. I. Early onset infection. *Am. J. Dis. Child.* 128:659–665, 1974.

8. Eisenfeld, L. et al. Systemic bacterial infections in neonatal deaths. *Am. J. Dis. Child.* 137:645–649, 1983.

9. Zipursky, A., and Jaber, H. M. The haematology of bacterial infection in newborn infants. *Clin. Haematol.* 7:175–193, 1978.

10. McCracken, G. H., Jr. Pharmacologic basis for antimicrobial therapy in newborn infants. *Am. J. Dis. Child.* 28:407–419, 1974.

11. Silverman, W. A. et al. A difference in mortality rate and incidence of kernicterus among premature infants allotted to two prophylactic antibacterial regimens. *Pediatrics* 18:614–624, 1956.

12. Wallman, I. S., and Hilton, H. B. Teeth pigmented by tetracycline. *Lancet* 1:827–829, 1962.

13. Cohlan, S. Q.; Bevelander, G.; and Tiamsic, T. Growth inhibition of prematures receiving tetracyclines. *Am. J. Dis. Child.* 105:453–461, 1963.

14. Weiss, C. F.; Glazko, A. J.; and Weston, J. K. Chloramphenicol in the newborn infant: a physiologic explanation of its toxicity when given in excessive doses. *N. Engl. J. Med.* 262:787–794, 1960.

15. Mauer, S. M.; Chavers, B. M.; and Kjellstrand, C. M. Treatment of an infant with severe chloramphenicol intoxication using charcoal-column hemoperfusion. *J. Pediatr.* 96:136–139, 1980.

16. Kessler, D. L., Jr.; Smith, A. L.; and Woodrum, D. E. Chloramphenicol toxicity in a neonate treated with exchange transfusion. *J. Pediatr.* 96:140–141, 1980.

17. Glazer, J. P. et al. Disposition of chloramphenicol in low birth weight infants. *Pediatrics* 66:573–578, 1980.

18. Rajchgot, P. et al. Initiation of chloramphenicol therapy in the newborn infant. *J. Pediatr.* 101:1018–1021, 1982.

19. Mulhall, A.; DeLouvois, J.; and Hurley, R. Efficacy of chloramphenicol in the treatment of neonatal and infantile meningitis: a study of 70 cases. *Lancet* 1:284–287, 1983.

20. Tessin, I. et al. Renal function of neonates during gentamicin treatment. *Arch. Dis. Child.* 57:758–760, 1982.

21. Szefler, S. J. et al. Relationship of gentamicin serum concentrations to gestational age in preterm and term neonates. *J. Pediatr.* 97:312–315, 1980.

22. Harris, M. C., and Polin, R. A. Neonatal septicemia. *Pediatr. Clin. North Am.* 30:243–258, 1983.

23. Hill, A.; Schackelford, G. D.; and Volpe, J. J. Ventriculitis with neonatal bacterial meningitis: identification by real-time ultrasound. *J. Pediatr.* 99:133–136, 1981.

24. Kairam, R., and DeVivo, D. C. Neurologic manifestations of congenital infection. *Clin. Perinatol.* 8:445–465, 1981.

25. Bell, W. E., and McGuiness, G. A. Suppurative central nervous system infections in the neonate. *Semin. Perinatol.* 6:1–24, 1982.

26. McCracken, G. H., Jrs., and Mize, S. G. A controlled study of intrathecal antibiotic therapy in gram-negative enteric meningitis of infancy: Report of the Neonatal Meningitis Co-operative Study Group. *J. Pediatr.* 89:66–72, 1976.

27. McCracken, G. H., Jr.; Mize, S. G.; and Threlkeld, N. Intraventricular gentamicin therapy in gram-negative bacillary meningitis of infancy: Report of the Second Neonatal Meningitis Co-operative Study Group. *Lancet* 1:787–791, 1980.

28. Lewis, B. R., and Gupta, J. M. Present prognosis in neonatal meningitis. *Med. J. Aust.* 1:695–697, 1977.

29. Eriksson, M. Neonatal septicemia. *Acta Paediatr. Scand.* 72:1–8, 1983.

30. Volpe, J. J. *Neurology of the newborn.* Philadelphia: W. B. Saunders Co., 1981, pp. 555–556.

31. Alfren, G. et al. Longterm follow-up of neonatal septicemia. *Acta Paediatr. Scand.* 67:769–773, 1978.

32. McCracken, G. H., Jr., and Feldman, W. E. Neonatal group B streptococcal infection (editorial). *J. Pediatr.* 89:203–204, 1976.

APPENDIX

Vermont Study, 1975–1980

Several laboratory tests suggested as helpful in diagnosing neonatal infection were evaluated, to determine which test or combination of tests was most helpful in confirming the presence of neonatal sepsis. Tests were chosen that (1) could provide a rapid result (preferably within an hour or less), (2) were simple, and (3) were relatively inexpensive. Such tests presumably could be available (or applicable) in any hospital in the world.

Subjects

All infants admitted to the intensive care nursery of the Medical Center Hospital of Vermont between October 1975 and March 1980 were eligible for entry into the study. Included in the study was any baby at risk for or suspected on clinical grounds of having sepsis or meningitis, who had had a sepsis work-up (including a blood culture).

Approximately 2000 infants were admitted to the intensive care nursery during the period of the study. Of these admissions, 524 babies were evaluated during the first week after birth, and 56 babies between 8 and 60 days of age also were investigated.

Designation of infection status had to be made retrospectively, as all babies were considered at risk for, or demonstrated clinical evidence

The results presented here were the basis of a thesis submitted for the degree of Doctor of Medicine at the University of Edinburgh. The degree was awarded in 1983.

of, sepsis. Those babies with positive blood and/or CSF and/or urine cultures within 48 hours of incubation were considered to have "proved" sepsis. Babies who received antibiotics for 3 days or less, and who survived (or died without evidence of infection at necropsy) were considered to be "not infected." A number of babies who had strong presumptive evidence of systemic infection (although blood and CSF cultures were negative) were considered to have "very probable" infection and were included with the proved cases as "infection" in other analyses.

Methods

Each infant who had a sepsis work-up had blood sent for aerobic and anaerobic cultures, and most had urine (suprapubic tap) and CSF fluid sent for culture. When indicated, a gastric aspirate was sent for smear to detect leukocytes or bacteria in babies evaluated early; a white blood cell (leukocyte) count and differential count were performed on all babies. Platelet estimates were performed on all babies, and when low or equivocal, a platelet count was performed. Samples for viral cultures were sent to a research laboratory within the university in any case where viral infection seemed likely. Chest radiographs were obtained in babies with associated respiratory signs.

An extra blood sample (0.5–1.0 ml) was taken for the following studies (after obtaining permission from a parent):

1. Immunoglobulin M (IgM) by gel radial immunodiffusion, and latex agglutination test
2. C-reactive protein (CRP) by latex agglutination text
3. Haptoglobin (Hp) by the Tarukoski method and latex agglutination test
4. Erythrocyte sedimentation rate (ESR) by microhematocrit capillary tube method (a so-called mini-ESR)
5. α_1-Acid glycoprotein (α_1-AGP) by gel radial immunodiffusion

The white blood cell count was performed with the Coulter counter and the differential counts by slide evaluation in the routine hematology laboratory.

Table 1.

Yield of Neonatal Sepsis Based on Investigation for Risk Factors (0–7 days after birth; usually investigated within 48 hours)*

Risk factors	Number investigated (n = 315)	Number with sepsis (n = 16)
Prolonged rupture of membranes ($>$24 hr)	140	8 (6%)
Preterm labor (unexplained)	113	7 (6%)
Maternal fever/infection	62	4 (6%)
Fetal tachycardia	4	1 (25%)
Meconium stained amniotic fluid (unexplained)	20	1 (5%)
Small for gestational age	28	0
Foul-smelling amniotic fluid	23	0
Prolonged labor ($>$24 hr)	1	0

*The numbers listed in tables 1 through 3 do not add up to the total because some babies were investigated for more than one reason.

At the end of approximately two and a half years (end of 1977), tests using IgM, α_1-AGP, and the Tarukoski evaluation of Hp were discontinued. The remaining tests, whose results could be obtained within an hour, were then applied at the bedside by the house staff and influenced their decisions about antibiotic use.

Comparisons of babies evaluated before (1975–1977, group 1) and after (1978–1980, group 2) tests were applied at the bedside were performed using chi-square analysis.

Analysis of babies of differing birth weights (above and below 2500 g) was performed using Student's t test.

Results

Of 524 babies investigated in the first week after birth, 298 were male and 226 were female (ratio of male to female = 1.3 : 1). There were 336 babies with birth weights of less than 2500 g and the same number were less than 37 weeks' gestation. Forty-one babies proved to have sepsis (23 males, 18 females, ratio male to female = 1.3 : 1) and 34 babies had "very probable" infection (20 males, 14 females, ratio male to female = 1.4 : 1). Of the 56 babies investigated after the first week

Table 2.

Yield of Neonatal Sepsis Based on Investigation for Clinical Factors in the Early Neonatal Period (0–7 days after birth)

Clinical factors	Number investigated (n = 283)	Number with sepsis (n = 35)
Lethargy	87	23 (26%)
Apnea (unexplained)	84	11 (13%)
Cyanotic spells (unexplained)	68	5 (7%)
Temperature instability	33	4 (12%)
Pustules	6	2 (33%)
Abdominal distention	13	2 (15%)
Convulsions/irritability	20	2 (10%)
Jaundice (unexplained)	21	2 (10%)
Poor feeding	21	1 (5%)
Petechiae/purpura	12	0
Hepatosplenomegaly	2	0

Table 3.

Yield of Neonatal Sepsis Based on Investigation for Clinical Factors in the Late Neonatal Period (8–60 days after birth)

Clinical factors	Number investigated (n = 56)	Number with sepsis (n = 12)
Lethargy	15	5 (33%)
Poor perfusion	5	3 (60%)
Convulsions/irritability	8	3 (38%)
Temperature instability	8	3 (38%)
Poor feeding	10	3 (30%)
Apnea	16	2 (13%)
Hepatosplenomegaly	1	1 (100%)
Diarrhea	2	1 (50%)
Cyanotic spells	5	1 (20%)
Abdominal distention	12	1 (8%)
Pustules	5	0
Jaundice	2	0

Table 4.
Distribution of Positive Tests at Initial Evaluation in Babies with Documented Sepsis in the Early Neonatal Period

Case no.	Age at SWU	Birth weight/ GA (g/ wk)	Sex	Positive culture	Causative organism	Survived/ died	ESR ≥15	WBC <5000	Latex CRP	I/T ratio ≥0.2	Latex Hp
1	3 days	2637/36	F	Blood	GBS	S		4300	+	0.50	−
2	1 day	1984/34	M	Blood	H. influenzae	S			+	0.34	−
3	2 days	2140/33	M	Blood	E. coli	S		4100	−	0.22	−
4	3 days	3126/37	F	Blood/ CSF	E. coli	S		4700	+		−
5	1 hr	2910/40	M	Blood	S. pneumoniae	S			+	0.34	−
6	4 hr	2240/35	M	Blood	B. subtilis	S			−	0.61	+
7	6 days	1000/28	F	Blood/ CSF	B. subtilis	D		(72,000)	−	0.44	+
8	3 days	3010/36	M	Blood/ CSF	E. coli	S	25	2200	+	0.46	−
9	2 days	2849/38	M	Blood/ CSF	GBS	S	27		+	0.65	−
10	1 day	1162/33	M	Blood	E. coli	D	(10)	2800	+	0.92	−
11	3 hr	1340/32	F	Blood	GBS	D	(10)	4600	−	0.31	
12	3 days	1520/31	M	Blood	E. coli	D			−		−
13	2 days	900/27	F	Blood	E. coli	D			−	0.23	−
14	4 hr	3700/40	M		Meningitis (? E. coli)‡	S	19		+	0.51	+

Table 4.
(continued)

Case no.	Age at SWU	Birth weight/GA (g/wk)	Sex	Positive culture	Causative organism	Survived/died	ESR ≥15	WBC <5000	Latex CRP	I/T ratio ≥0.2	Latex Hp
15	4 days	1180/28	M	Blood	GBS*	S	20	1600	+	+	+
16	1 day	2665/35	M	Blood	GBS	D		1500	−	1.0†	−
17	7 days	2098/35	F	Blood	E. coli	S	33	3200	+	0.47	+
18	2 days	1740/31	F	Blood	GBS	D		1800	−	1.0†	−
19	3 days	2000/36	M	Blood	E. coli	S	25	3700	+	0.24	+
20	6 days	2420/44	F	Blood/CSF	E. coli	S			+	0.44	+
21	14 hr	1400/32	F	Blood	GBS	D		1400	−	1.0†	−
22	2 days	2948/40	M	Blood	GBS	S		2800	−	0.86	−
23	6 days	2900/40	F	Blood/CSF	E. coli	S	32		−	0.21	+
24	6 hr	2360/36	F	Blood	GBS	D		3400	−	0.58	−
25	5 days	1550/33	F	Blood/CSF	GBS*	S			+	0.25	−
26	5 days	3000/40	M	Blood/CSF	GBS	S	22		−	0.30	−
27	7 days	5960/40	M	Blood	E. coli*	S	15		−	0.32	−
28	1 hr	1210/31	F	Blood	E. coli	S			−	0.52	+

29	1 hr	2960/40	F	Blood	GBS	S			+	0.48	−
30	3 days	1810/34	M	Blood	Staph. aureus	S		2800	−	0.37	−
31	2 hr	2460/36	M	Blood/CSF	GBS	D			−	0.33	−
32	1 day	2790/37	M	Blood	GDS	S	25		+	0.39	−
33	12 hr	2800/37	M	Blood	Campylobacter jejuni	S	(10)		−	0.58	+
34	10 hr	3780/40	F	Blood	E. coli	ɔ			+	0.26	+
35	2 days	2820/36	M	Blood	E. coli	S		3200	+		−
36	7 days	680/28	M	Blood	Staph. epidermidis	S		(36,700)	+	0.25	−
37	5 days	2580/37	F	Blood/CSF	Proteus spp.	S	22		+		+
38	10 hr	1460/31	M	Blood	GBS	S		2500	−	1.0†	−
39	3 hr	1080/30	M	Urine	E. coli	S	(10)	4600	−		−
40	6 days	1370/33	F	Blood/CSF	E. coli	S		3500	−	0.35	−
41	5 days	1100/31	F	Blood	Staph. aureus	S			+		+

NOTE: ESR = erythrocyte sedimentation rate; GA = gestational age; GBS = group B β-hemolytic streptococci; GDS = group D β-hemolytic streptococci; I/T ratio = immature to total neutrophil ratio; latex CRP = C-reactive protein latex agglutination test; latex Hp = haptoglobin latex agglutination test; SWU = sepsis work-up; WBC = white blood cell count.

*Had negative cultures and tests shortly after birth.

†1–2 bands; 0 polymorphonuclear leukocytes.

‡On the basis of CSF cell count, glucose, and Gram stain.

Table 5.

Distribution of Positive Tests at Initial Evaluation in Babies with "Very Probable" Infection in the Early Neonatal Period

Case no.	Age at SWU	Birth weight/ GA (g/wk)	Sex	Factors suggesting infection	ESR ≥15	WBC <5000	Latex CRP	I/T ratio ≥0.2	Latex Hp
1	2 days	3544/40	M	Pneumonia*			+		+
2	8 hr	2041/35	M	Maternal GBS, pneumonia		2300	–	0.33	–
3	2 hr	1956/36	M	Petechiae and purpura; *S. aureus* in CSF at 3 days†			+	0.83	–
4	12 hr	2840/40	M	Lethargy; tracheal aspirate: GBS			+	0.42	–
5	2 days	4111/41	M	Fever, pustule grew *S. aureus*		(24,600)	+	(0.18)	–
6	4 days	2280/35	M	Poor feeding; shock; response to antibiotics	25	3200	–	(0.16)	–
7	2 hr	1300/32	M	PROM; maternal infection and antibiotics; lethargy	17		–	0.41	–
8	2 days	2060/38	F	Pneumonia; tracheal aspirate: GBS		3800	+	0.48	–

9	4 hr	2980/40	F	Apnea; shock; antibiotics prior to blood culture	17		+	0.65	−
10	6 hr	3232/40	F	Fever; maternal GBS	(14)	(40,600)	+	0.59	+
11	4 hr	4000/38	M	Maternal fever; tracheal aspirate: E. coli; antibiotics prior to culture		(29,000)	+	(0.15)	−
12	3 days	2395/39	M	Pneumonia; fever	27		+	0.25	+
13	1 hr	1630/33	M	PROM 48 hr; pneumonia			−	(0.16)	−
14	1 hr	1970/34	F	PROM; pneumonia			−	0.43	−
15	2 hr	2250/36	F	PROM 48 hr; pneumonia; gram-pos. rod at 10 d (blood culture)†			+	0.21	−
16	1 hr	1210/28	M	PROM 2 wk; Apgars $1^1/1^5$		4000	+	(0.17)	−
17	1 hr	1480/30	F	PROM 4 wk; foul-smelling amniotic fluid; maternal fever and antibiotic therapy; pneumonia			+	0.50	−

Table 5.
(continued)

Case no.	Age at SWU	Birth weight/ GA (g/wk)	Sex	Factors suggesting infection	ESR ≥ 5	WBC < 5000	Latex CRP	I/T ratio ≥ 0.2	Latex Hp
18	4 hr	3440/40	F	Apnea; pneumonia with pleural effusion			+	0.24	–
19	2 days	3060/40	M	Apnea; lethargy; pneumonia			+		+
20	2 hr	2180/34	M	PROM; pneumonia	(10)		+	0.22	–
21	0	2830/37	F	Respiratory difficulty; pneumonia		(30,200)	–		–
22	0	1400/30	M	PROM; pneumonia; old pleuritis at necropsy; pos. buffy coat smear		3200	+	0.39	–
23	12 hr	930/29	M	Maternal fever; foul-smelling amniotic fluid; apnea	26		–	0.75	–
24	1 day	4100/38	M	Pneumonia; fever			–	0.82	+
25	2 days	3550/40	F	Lymphangitis		(32,200)	+	(0.18)	+

26	1 hr	2440/35	F	Maternal UTI; premature labor; pneumonia		+	0.45	−
27	1 day	2520/36	F	Respiratory difficulty; irritable; pneumonia		+		+
28	2 hr	3860/40	M	PROM; foul-smelling amniotic fluid; pneumonia		+	0.66	−
29	1 hr	780/28	M	PROM 72 hr; pneumonia	30	+	0.24	−
30	1 hr	1240/31	F	PROM 72 hr; maternal culture: GBS; pneumonia	15	+	0.43	−
31	3 days	1940/35	F	Premature labor; pneumonia; endotracheal aspirate: E. coli	(13)	+	0.80	−
32	1 day	1930/34	F	Maternal UTI; PROM 48 hr; foul-smelling amniotic fluid; CSF: Bacillus sp. (broth)†	17	+	0.40	−

Table 5.
(continued)

Case no.	Age at SWU	Birth weight/ GA (g/wk)	Sex	Factors suggesting infection	ESR ≥15	WBC <5000	Latex CRP	I/T ratio ≥0.2	Latex Hp
33	1 day	1780/33	M	Premature labor; PROM; pneumonia; amniotic fluid: GBS		4700	+	0.40	—
34	1 day	760/29	M	Maternal fever; apnea; placenta: GBS	28		+	0.32	—

NOTE: ESR = erythrocyte sedimentation rate; GA = gestational age; GBS = group B β-hemolytic streptococci; I/T ratio = immature to total neutrophil ratio; latex CRP = C = reactive protein latex agglutination test; Hp = haptoglobin latex agglutination test; PROM = prolonged rupture of membranes (≥24hr.); SWU = sepsis work-up; WBC = white blood cell count.

*Pneumonia indicates radiographic infiltrates consistent with this diagnosis.

†Considered to be contaminant organism.

Table 6.

Laboratory Data at Initial Evaluation for Infants with Proved Sepsis in the Late Neonatal Period

Patient No./Sex	Birth weight (g)	Gestational age (wk)	Age at evaluation (days)	Causative organism	Source	WBC count <5.0 (×10⁹/l)	I/T ratio ≥0.2	Latex CRP	Latex Hp	Mini-ESR ≥15 (mm/hr)
1/M	3410	40	20	Staphylococcus aureus	Blood	(32.9)		−	+	
2/M	3487	40	9	Group A streptococcus	Blood	(27.2)	0.2	−	+	17
3/M	780	33	58	Enterobacter	Blood	4.9	0.32	+	−	42
4/M	2180	35	13	S. aureus	Blood	(24.9)		+	−	
5/F*	690	33	13	Escherichia coli	Blood		0.4	+	−	
6/M	2268	40	21	S. aureus	Blood, central venous catheter		0.21	+	−	25
7/F	750	32	9	S. epidermidis	Blood	3.8		+	−	
8/F	3390	38	33	E. coli	Blood, urine			+	−	30
9/M*	4280	40	18	Group B streptococcus	Blood, CSF	4.0	0.58	+	−	
10/M	3720	40	47	Haemophilus influenzae	Blood, CSF	3.9	0.77	+	−	
11/M	780	28	12	Group D streptococcus	Urine			−	+	25
12/M	2700	37	13	Pseudomonas aeruginosa	Blood		0.49	+	−	20

NOTE: See table 5 for explanation of abbreviations.

*Died.

Table 7.

Predictive Value for Sepsis of Several Leukocyte Levels Suggested as Indicative of Neonatal Infection, at Different Ages During the First Week after Birth

	Days after birth											Total	
	0		1		2		3–4		5–7					
Total evaluated	296		110		40		50		28				524	
Number with proved sepsis	8	(3%)	9	(8%)	7	(18%)	7	(14%)	10	(36%)			41	(8%)
Leukocytes														
$\geq 20.0 \times 10^9$/l	0/50		0/27		0/5		0/1		2/6	(33%)			2/89*	(2%)
$\geq 25.0 \times 10^9$/l	0/24		0/9		0/2		0/0		2/2	(100%)			2/37	(5%)
$\geq 30.0 \times 10^9$/l	0/11		0/3		0/1		0/0		2/2	(100%)			2/17	(12%)
$< 10.0 \times 10^9$/l	6/93	(6%)	7/40	(18%)	6/22	(27%)	7/34	(21%)	4/11	(36%)			30/200	(15%)
$< 5.0 \times 10^9$/l	2/16	(13%)	5/10	(50%)	5/7	(71%)	5/13	(38%)	2/2	(100%)			19/48	(40%)
$< 4.0 \times 10^9$/l	0/5		5/7	(71%)	4/6	(67%)	3/8	(38%)	2/2	(100%)			14/28	(50%)
Neutrophils														
$> 10.0 \times 10^9$/l	0/79		0/44		0/11		0/5		3/9	(33%)			3/148	(2%)
$> 15.0 \times 10^9$/l	0/24		0/14		0/5				2/3	(67%)			2/45	(4%)
$< 1.5 \times 10^9$/l	3/21	(14%)	3/8	(38%)	3/3	(100%)	2/8	(25%)	2/3	(67%)			13/43	(30%)
$< 1.0 \times 10^9$/l	3/12	(35%)	3/6	(50%)	2/2	(100%)	2/6	(33%)	1/1	(100%)			11/27	(41%)

Immature neutrophils											
> 1.5 × 10⁹/l	1/56	(2%)	4/39	(10%)	1/7	(14%)	0/6		4/5	(80%)	10/113 (9%)
> 1.0 × 10⁹/l	4/82	(5%)	4/52	(8%)	1/10	(10%)	1/8	(13%)	5/6	(83%)	15/158 (9%)
Immature/total neutrophil ratio											
≥ 0.15	7/82	(9%)	9/56	(16%)	6/18	(33%)	6/16	(38%)	8/9	(89%)	36/181 (20%)
≥ 0.20	7/63	(11%)	9/45	(20%)	6/12	(50%)	4/11	(36%)	8/9	(89%)	34/140 (24%)
≥ 0.30	7/41	(17%)	6/28	(21%)	4/7	(57%)	2/6	(33%)	6/6	(100%)	25/88 (28%)

*By providing the individual numbers, the values for sensitivity and specificity can be derived. For example, from 2/89 we know that sensitivity is 2/41 (5%) and specificity is 396/483 (82%).

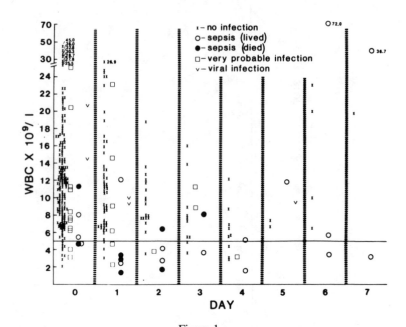

Figure 1.

The total leukocyte count at the time of initial evaluation for sepsis is shown in infants with birth weight less than 2500 g, according to infection status at different times of evaluation.

of birth, the distribution was 37 boys, 19 girls, and 34 low birth weight infants, with 12 proved cases of sepsis (9 boys, 3 girls). (See tables 1–6 for further details.)

Leukocyte Count

By careful perusal of table 7, it can be seen that some values are more sensitive than others, but lose something either in specificity or predictive value. The most useful levels seem to be total leukocyte count of $< 5.0 \times 10^9/l$ (sensitivity 19/41, 46%; positive predictive value 19/48, 40%) and an immature to total (I/T) neutrophil ratio of ≥ 0.2 (sensitivity 34/41, 83%; positive predictive value 34/140, 24%). It is evident,

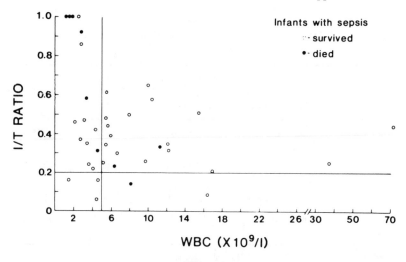

Figure 2.
The immature to total (I/T) neutrophil ratio is plotted against the total leukocyte count in infants with proved sepsis during the first week after delivery.

however, that a total leukocyte count of $< 10.0 \times 10^9/l$ and an I/T ratio of ≥ 0.15 seem to be the most sensitive indicators (30/41, 73% and 36/41, 88% respectively), without losing too much in specificity. Elevated leukocyte counts only seem to be of value at the end of the first week. Figure 1 shows the values for total leukocyte counts according to infection status by day of age of evaluation in low birth weight infants. In Figure 2 infants with proved sepsis are plotted by WBC and I/T ratio.

When noninfected infants with birth weights above and below 2500 grams were compared, the low birth weight infants had significantly lower levels of total leukocytes, segmented neutrophils, and immature neutrophils, but the I/T ratio was not affected (table 8).

Erythrocyte Sedimentation Rate

Results of the mini-ESR for different groups of babies (proved sepsis, very probable infection, and not infected) are provided in table 9 according to the day of evaluation. Figure 3 shows the distribution of values in low birth weight infants according to infection status by day of age at evaluation.

Table 8.

Mean (± SEM) Values for Various Leukocyte Counts in Noninfected Infants with Birth Weights Above and Below 2500 g

Age	Test (× 10⁹/l)	Birth weight <2500 g (n = 218)	Birth weight >2500 g (n = 143)	*p* Value (*t* test)
0–7 days	Total WBC count	11.6 ± 0.43	17.3 ± 0.59	<0.001
	Segmented neutrophils	5.2 ± 0.27	9.9 ± 0.43	<0.001
	Band neutrophils	0.76 ± 0.09	1.5 ± 0.15	<0.001
	Immature/total neutrophil ratio	0.12 ± 0.01	0.13 ± 0.01	NS

NS = not significant.

Table 9.

Erythrocyte Sedimentation Rate (ESR) by Day of Evaluation and Infection Status

			ESR (Mean ± SEM)			
Age	n	Not infected	n	Very probable infection	n	Proved sepsis
0–6 hours	272	1.9 ± 0.2	16	6.4 ± 2.1	8	7.4 ± 2.1
1 day	90	2.5 ± 0.3	11	10.9 ± 2.8	9	6.8 ± 2.5
2 days	29	1.7 ± 0.2	4	6.5 ± 1.0	7	6.1 ± 3.6
3–4 days	40	3.7 ± 0.5	3	22.0 ± 7.0	7	12.6 ± 4.8
5–7 days	18	6.4 ± 2.0	0		10	14.7 ± 4.7
Total (0–7 days)	449	2.3 ± 0.2	34	9.2 ± 1.6	41	9.7 ± 1.5

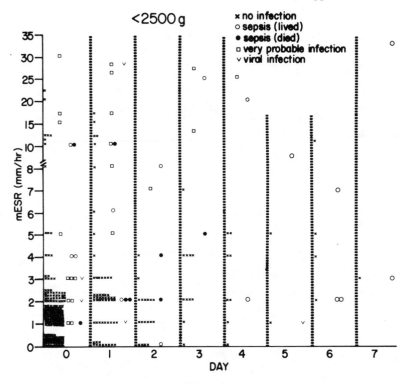

Figure 3.
The distribution of mini-ESR values in low birth weight infants is shown according to infection status by day of age at evaluation.

C-Reactive Protein

The CRP latex agglutination test provides semiquantitative results, therefore, it is not possible to plot the levels in the same way as leukocytes and ESR. Table 10 shows the frequency of positive tests by day of evaluation according to infection status.

Haptoglobin

The modified Hp latex agglutination test shows a positive result at levels greater than 25 mg/dl. In older infants (8–60 days) the Hp latex agglutination test was positive at levels greater than 50 mg/dl. Table 11 shows the frequency of positive tests by day of evaluation according to infection status.

Table 10.

Frequency of Positive Latex C-Reactive Protein Tests by Day of Evaluation and Infection Status

Age	Not infected	Very probable infection	Proved sepsis	Total
0–6 hours	17	12	4	33
1 day	17	8	5	30
2 days	2	4	2	8
3–4 days	6	2	6	14
5–7 days	3	0	5	8
Total 0–7 days	45	26	22	93
8–30 days	4	3	6	13
31–60 days	3	3	3	9
Total	52	32	31	115

Table 11.

Frequency of Positive Latex Haptoglobin Tests by Day of Evaluation and Infection Status

Age	Not infected	Very probable infection	Proved sepsis	Total
0–6 hours	7	0	3	10
1 day	4	4	2	10
2 days	1	2	0	3
3–4 days	3	1	3	7
5–7 days	1	0	6	7
Total 0–7 days	16	7	14	37
8–30 days	4	2	3	9
31–60 days	0	1	0	1
Total	20	10	17	47

Table 12.
Levels of α_1-Acid Glycoprotein (mean ± SEM) in mg/dl at Various Ages During the First Week After Delivery According to Infection Status

Age	n	Not infected	n	Very probable infection	n	Proved sepsis
0–6 hours	125	23 ± 1.6	4	77 ± 11.0	4	65 ± 18
1 day	72	25 ± 2.3	3	71 ± 16.0	4	32 ± 12
2 days	20	29 ± 4.2	3	63 ± 2.4	5	35 ± 10
3–4 days	20	41 ± 4.0	2	134 ± 27.0	6	83 ± 14
5–7 days	7	50 ± 11.0	0		3	129 ± 44

α_1-Acid Glycoprotein

The results of α_1-AGP levels in the first 278 babies are presented in table 12 according to age and infection status. The infected groups have significantly higher levels ($p < 0.0001$) than the noninfected group, when all ages are combined. The survivors of sepsis (n = 14) had a mean α_1-AGP level of 90 mg/dl, whereas those who died of sepsis (n = 7) had a mean α_1-AGP level of 19 mg/dl. Three babies died on day 1 with α_1-AGP levels of 34, 15, and 13 mg/dl, respectively, and two infants died on day 2 with respective levels of 30 and 14 mg/dl. One other baby who subsequently died had an initial level of 48 mg/dl.

In figure 4 the α_1-AGP values obtained in the first 24 hours after delivery are plotted against gestational age, according to infection status. There was a statistically significant correlation between gestational age and levels of α_1-AGP in the not infected group ($r = 0.452, p < 0.001$).

Tests of Limited Value

In the first half of the study, platelet counts and IgM levels were routinely evaluated and gastric aspirate smears were examined when indicated.

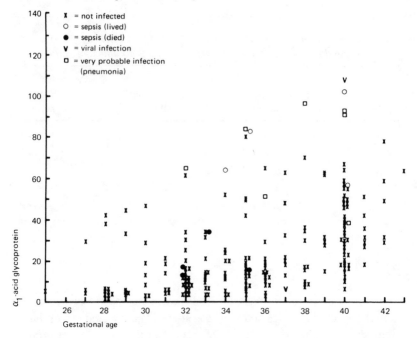

Figure 4.
The levels of α₁-acid glycoprotein (in mg/dl) are plotted against gestational age for all babies evaluated within 24 hours of delivery. Levels above 50 mg/dl are considered abnormal at this age.

Platelet Count

Platelet counts $< 150 \times 10^9/l$ were considered abnormal. There were very few abnormal counts when the babies were first evaluated. Indeed, only 15 babies had abnormal counts and only 2 were found to have sepsis. A number of babies did develop low platelet counts later in their course.

Immunoglobulin M Levels

A level exceeding 0.3 g/l was considered abnormal, as this was the limit for the latex reagent (designed to detect abnormal levels). Of 45 infants with an IgM level > 0.3 g/l (using radial immunodiffusion), only 3 infants proved to have sepsis.

Gastric Aspirate Smear

A total of 101 babies had gastric contents aspirated and sent for smear. The presence of five or more polymorphonuclear leukocytes per high-power field was considered abnormal. Twenty babies had positive smears, four of whom were infected. Of 81 babies with negative smears, 4 were infected. These findings were not significant (x^2 with Yates correction = 3.14; $p > 0.05$).

Combinations of Tests

Details of sensitivity, specificity, predictive value, and efficiency are provided in table 13 for five individual tests and two combinations. Details are provided for both sepsis and "infection" detection, in babies evaluated during the first week after birth.

One might suspect that increased predictive value would be obtained with an increasing number of tests positive. This is suggested in table 14, but the numbers with multiple tests positive are small.

Because not all tests may be available, it may be useful to know the predictiveness of various combinations. These are provided in tables 15 and 16.

In a few cases, sequential measurements were carried out. Repeat studies were carried out on seven babies approximately 24 hours after initial evaluation. The results are presented in table 17 and show that in four cases the CRP initially was negative but became positive within 24 hours. The ESR was more erratic, with minimal increases in two infants (who died) and a decrease in another. In three infants who survived, there was a brisk increase in the leukocyte count.

Possible Amniotic Fluid Infection

Of a total of 276 babies investigated for prolonged rupture of membranes (> 24 hours), maternal fever/infection, and/or unexplained pre-

Table 13.

*Sensitivity, Specificity, Predictive Value, and Efficiency of Several Tests for Sepsis and Infection**

	Sensitivity $\left(\dfrac{a}{a+c}\right)$		Specificity $\left(\dfrac{d}{b+d}\right)$		Positive predictive value $\left(\dfrac{a}{a+b}\right)$		Negative predictive value $\left(\dfrac{d}{c+d}\right)$		Efficiency $\left(\dfrac{a+d}{a+b+c+d}\right)$	
Sepsis										
I/T ratio ≥ 0.2	34/41	(83%)	376/483	(78%)	34/141	(24%)	376/383	(98%)	410/524	(78%)
WBC count < 5.0×10^9/l	19/41	(46%)	453/483	(94%)	19/49	(39%)	453/475	(95%)	472/524	(90%)
Positive CRP latex agglutination test	22/41	(54%)	412/483	(85%)	22/93	(24%)	412/431	(96%)	434/524	(83%)
Positive Hp latex agglutination test	14/41	(34%)	460/483	(95%)	14/37	(38%)	460/487	(94%)	474/524	(90%)
ESR ≥ 15 mm/hr	11/41	(27%)	464/483	(96%)	11/29	(38%)	464/494	(94%)	475/524	(91%)
Any two or more tests	38/41	(93%)	422/483	(87%)	38/99	(38%)	422/426	(99%)	460/524	(88%)

I/T ratio ≥ 0.2 + WBC count < 5.0	38/41	(93%)	359/483	(74%)	38/162	(23%)	359/362	(99%)	397/524	(76%)
Infection*										
I/T ratio ≥ 0.2	59/75	(79%)	367/449	(82%)	59/141	(42%)	367/387	(95%)	426/524	(81%)
WBC count < 5.0 × 10^9/l	25/75	(33%)	425/449	(95%)	25/49	(51%)	425/475	(89%)	450/524	(86%)
Positive CRP latex agglutination test	48/75	(64%)	404/449	(90%)	48/93	(52%)	404/431	(94%)	452/524	(86%)
Positive Hp latex agglutination test	21/75	(28%)	433/449	(96%)	21/37	(57%)	433/487	(89%)	454/524	(87%)
ESR ≥ 15 mm/hr	20/75	(27%)	439/449	(98%)	20/29	(69%)	439/494	(89%)	459/524	(88%)
Any two or more tests	67/75	(89%)	417/449	(93%)	67/99	(68%)	417/426	(98%)	484/524	(92%)
I/T ratio ≥ 0.2 + WBC count < 5.0	64/75	(85%)	351/449	(78%)	64/162	(40%)	351/362	(97%)	415/524	(79%)

NOTE: Incidence of sepsis is 41/524 (7.8%), incidence of infection is 75/524 (14.3%).

*Infection = proved sepsis group plus very probable infection group.

Table 14.

Sepsis Screen Scores for Infants Evaluated in the First Week

	Score of sepsis screen* No. (%)				
	0–1	2	3	4	5
Sepsis	3 (1)	24 (34)	8 (39)	4 (67)	2 (100)
Viral infection	3 (1)	3 (4)	1 (5)	0	0
Very probable infection	5 (1)	19 (28)	9 (43)	1 (17)	0
Not infected	415 (97)	23 (33)	3 (14)	1 (17)	0
Total	426	69	21	6	2

*The score is derived from the presence of five diagnostic findings: WBC count $< 5.0 \times 10^9/$l; immature/total neutrophil ratio > 0.2; ESR $\geqslant 15$ mm/hr; positive CRP latex agglutination test; and positive Hp latex agglutination test.

Table 15.

Predictive Value of Different Pairs of Tests for Sepsis in the Early Neonatal Period (0–7 days after birth)

Combination of tests	Total positive	Positive score proved infection	Positive predictive accuracy (%)	False-positives*
WBC and I/T ratio	22	15	68	3
CRP and I/T ratio	50	15	30	10
Hp and I/T ratio	18	10	56	2
ESR and I/T ratio	21	9	43	2
WBC and CRP	14	9	64	1
ESR and CRP	19	8	42	2
Hp and CRP	22	8	36	3
Hp and ESR	9	6	67	0
WBC and ESR	5	4	80	1
WBC and Hp	5	3	60	2
Any two or more	99	38/41 (93%)	38/99 (38%)	27/442 (6%)

*Includes positive combination in the not infected group; excludes very probable infection group.

Table 16.

Predictive Value of Different Pairs of Tests for Sepsis in the Late Neonatal Period (8–60 days after birth)

Combination of tests	Total positive	Positive score proved infection	Positive predictive accuracy (%)	False-positives*
CRP and I/T ratio	10	6	60	2
WBC and CRP	6 (+2)†	4 (+1)	67 (63%)	1
ESR and CRP	8	4	50	1
ESR and I/T ratio	7	4	57	1
WBC and I/T ratio	6 (+2)	3 (+1)	50 (50%)	1
Hp and ESR	3	2	67	0
WBC and ESR	3 (+1)	1 (+1)	33 (50%)	1
Hp and I/T ratio	2	1	50	0
WBC and Hp	0 (+5)	0 (+2)	— (40%)	0 (+1)
Hp and CRP	2	0	0	0
Any two or more	23 (+3)	10 (+2)	43 (46%)	2 (+1)
% of total (n = 56)	41% (46%)	83% (100%)		4% (5%)

*Excludes "very probable" group.

†Figures in parentheses indicate the addition of WBC count $\geq 20.0 \times 10^9/l$.

term labor, only 6% proved to have sepsis. Of 150 babies evaluated for a single risk factor, only 2 proved to have sepsis, compared with 13 of 126 babies with multiple factors for investigation ($x^2 = 10.93$, $p < 0.001$).

Conclusions

While the combination of tests described here cannot be considered infallible, these tests seem to provide the most reliable indicators of infection so far described. It will be important to evaluate them in other centers, particularly where other organisms are more prevalent. By

Table 17.
Sequential Values of Several Tests in 7 Infants with Proved Sepsis

Case no.	Birth weight (g)	Sex	Day of pos. SWU	Organism	Initial values					Values 16–24 hr. later				Survived/ died
					WBC	I/T ratio	ESR	Latex CRP		WBC	I/T ratio	ESR	Latex CRP	
24	2360	F	1	GBS	3.4	0.58	2	−		8.4	0.38	3	+	D
26	3000	M	5	GBS	6.7	0.30	22	−		25.6	0.21	12	+	S
29	2960	F	0	GBS	5.5	0.48	2	+		23.5	0.30	17	+	S
31	2460	M	0	GBS	11.3	0.33	1	−		13.7	0.49	6	+	D
33	2800	M	1	CJ	10.4	0.58	10	+		11.7	0.05	38	+	S
39	1080	M	0	E. coli	4.6	0.06	10	+		6.9	0	22	+	S
40	1370	F	6	E. coli	3.5	0.37	2	−		15.1	0.08	15	+	S

NOTE: CJ = *Campylobacter jejuni*; GBS = group B β-hemolytic streptococcus; SWU = sepsis work-up.

combining the leukocyte count with the measurement of acute-phase protein levels, one may be getting the "best of both worlds."

Although these tests are nonspecific indicators of infection, the simplicity of the tests and the rapidity with which the results can be obtained mean that they (1) could be available in almost any hospital where babies are delivered, (2) could help to make an early diagnosis of neonatal sepsis, and (3) could be incorporated into decisions about whether or not to start antibiotics. In this investigation, the tests were accepted as valuable by house officers and a decrease in antibiotic use resulted. This was most pronounced when a single risk factor (e.g., prolonged rupture of membranes) was the reason for investigation.

No single test can be considered entirely satisfactory, but the single most useful test seems to be the I/T ratio. Unlike some other tests, it does not seem to be influenced by birth weight or gestational age. When the I/T ratio (or fraction) was > 0.2, 34 of 41 infants with sepsis, aged 0 to 7 days, were detected (sensitivity = 83%), and 7 of 12 (58%) infants between the ages of 8 and 60 days were detected, but positive predictive accuracy (i.e., number of proved cases with a positive test/ total positive tests) was only 24% and 40%, respectively. In contrast, a combination of tests designated as a "sepsis screen" (2 or more of 5 diagnostic findings: WBC count < $5.0 \times 10^9/l$, I/T ratio ≥ 0.2 ESR ≥ 15 mm/hr, positive CRP latex agglutination test, and positive Hp latex agglutination test) detected 38 of 41 infants with sepsis in the first week after birth (sensitivity = 93%) and 10 of 12 infants (83%) aged between 8 and 60 days. Positive predictive accuracy for the sepsis screen was 38% (0–7 days) and 43% (8–60 days). When infection (defined as sepsis group plus very probable infection group) was evaluated, sensitivity of the sepsis screen was 89% and positive predictive accuracy was 68% for infants aged 0 to 7 days. The most useful pair of tests in the first week after birth was WBC count < $5.0 \times 10^9/l$ and I/T ratio ≥ 0.2, which detected 15 of 41 (37%) infants with sepsis with a positive predictive accuracy of 68% for sepsis and 86% for infection. Between 8 and 60 days, the best pair of tests was positive CRP latex agglutination test and I/T ratio ≥ 0.2, with 6 of 12 (50%) infants with sepsis detected and positive predictive accuracy of 60% for sepsis and 80% for infection.

INDEX